complete cookery

Diabetic

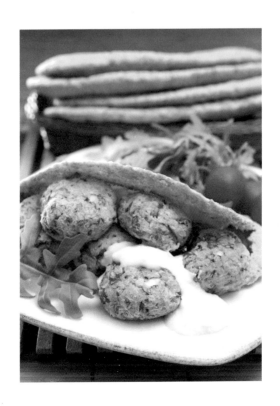

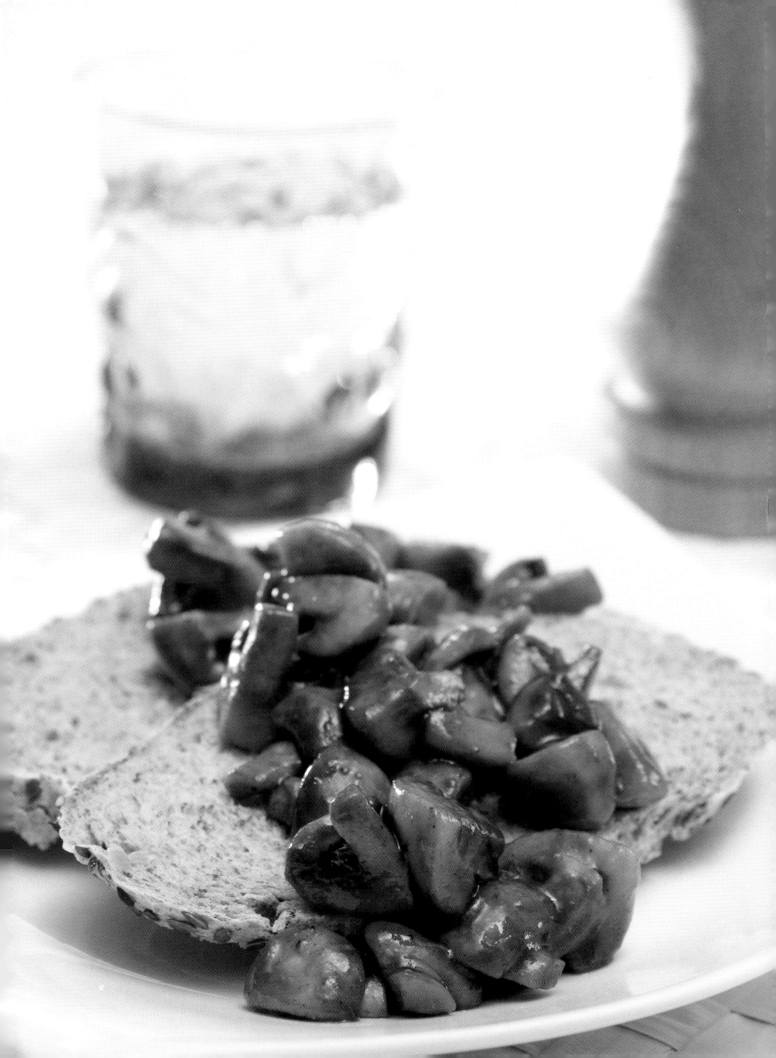

complete cookery

Diabetic

Jacqueline Bellefontaine

Published by SILVERDALE BOOKS
An imprint of Bookmart Ltd
Registered number 2372865
Trading as Bookmart Ltd
Blaby Road
Wigston
Leicester LE18 4SE

© 2006 D&S Books Ltd

D&S Books Ltd
Kerswell,
Parkham Ash, Bideford
Devon, England
EX39 5PR

e-mail us at:- enquiries@d-sbooks.co.uk

ISBN   10 – 1-84509-440-9
          13 – 9-781-84509-440-9

DS0135. Complete Cookery: Diabetic

Creative Director: Sarah King
Project Editor: Claire Bone
Designer: Debbie Fisher
Photographer: Colin Bowling/Paul Forrester

Fonts: New York, Helvetica and Bradley Hand

Material from this book previously appeared 100 great recipes: Diabetic.

Printed in Thailand

1 3 5 7 9 10 8 6 4 2

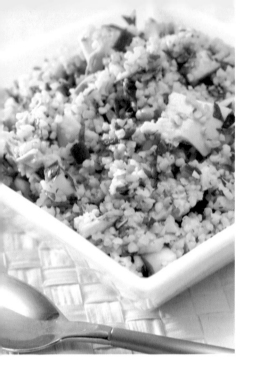

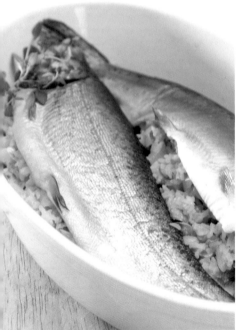

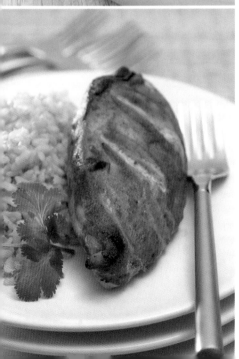

Contents

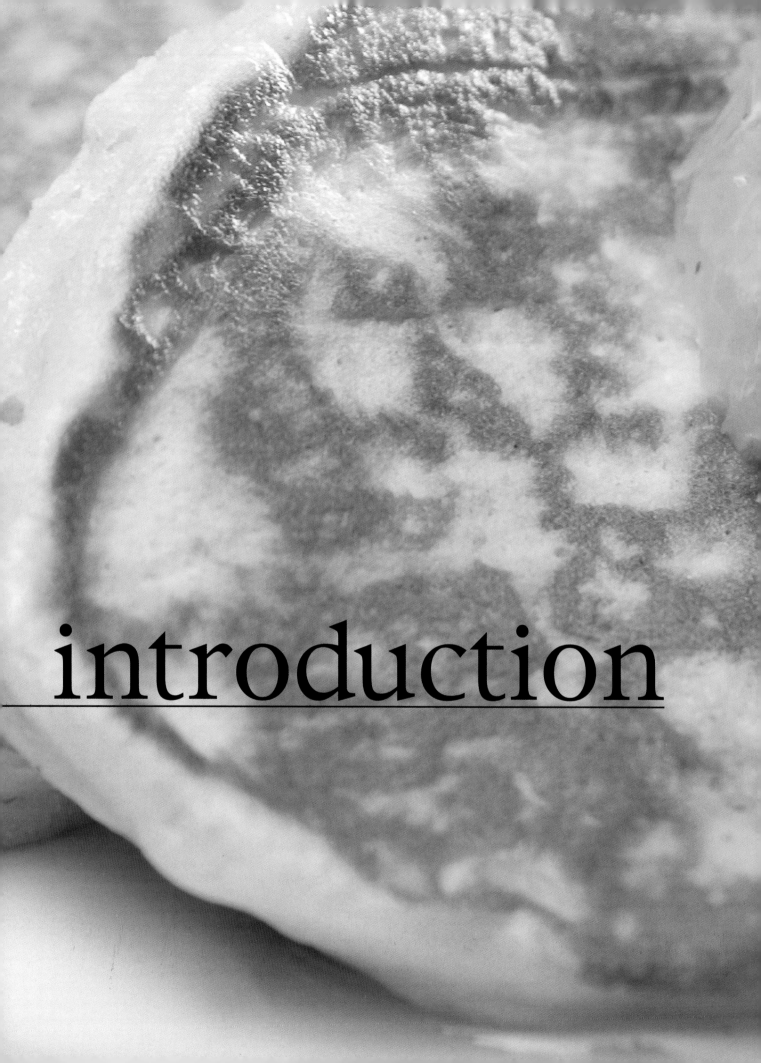

introduction

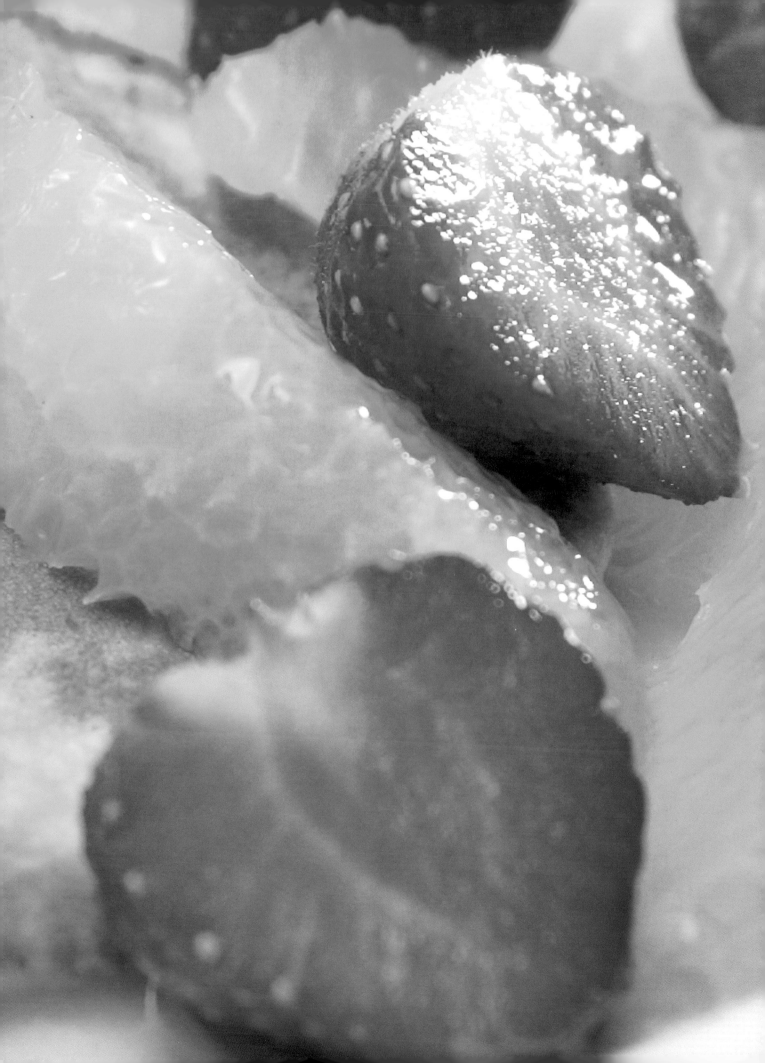

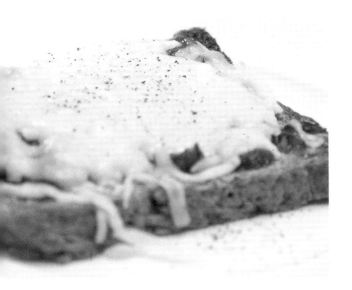

Whether you have had diabetes all your life, have recently been diagnosed, or simply know someone who has diabetes and want to cook for them, buying this cook book is a good start. As you will no doubt be aware, diet plays a very important role in the management of diabetes, and by doing your own cooking you take control of your diet. Convenience foods are all too often loaded with hidden sugar or fat or both, but by cooking meals and dishes from scratch you know exactly what is in the food you are eating and can make informed decisions on how to manage your diet.

Most people with diabetes will have to make changes to their diet. These will be life-long changes, so if you have recently been diagnosed be careful of making sudden radical changes which you may then find difficult to stick to. For example, start increasing the fibre in your diet by eating wholemeal bread, then introduce wholemeal pasta and brown rice, and finally use wholemeal flour in your baking. Introduce beans and pulses into your diet if you haven't already done so. Start by making one meal a week based on beans and pulses and gradually increase the number of meals. Make sure that you eat at least five portions of fruit and vegetables a day. Base your meals around carbohydrates such as potatoes, rice, pasta, bread, beans and pulses. Remember, low fat and low sugar are key to a diet for people with diabetes.

Most people with diabetes are overweight. Losing weight and keeping fat intake down can play a very significant part in diabetes management. Losing weight can help to control blood glucose levels. Following a calorie-controlled diet and increasing exercise will help weight loss.

ALWAYS FOLLOW THE ADVICE OF YOUR HEALTH CARE TEAM.

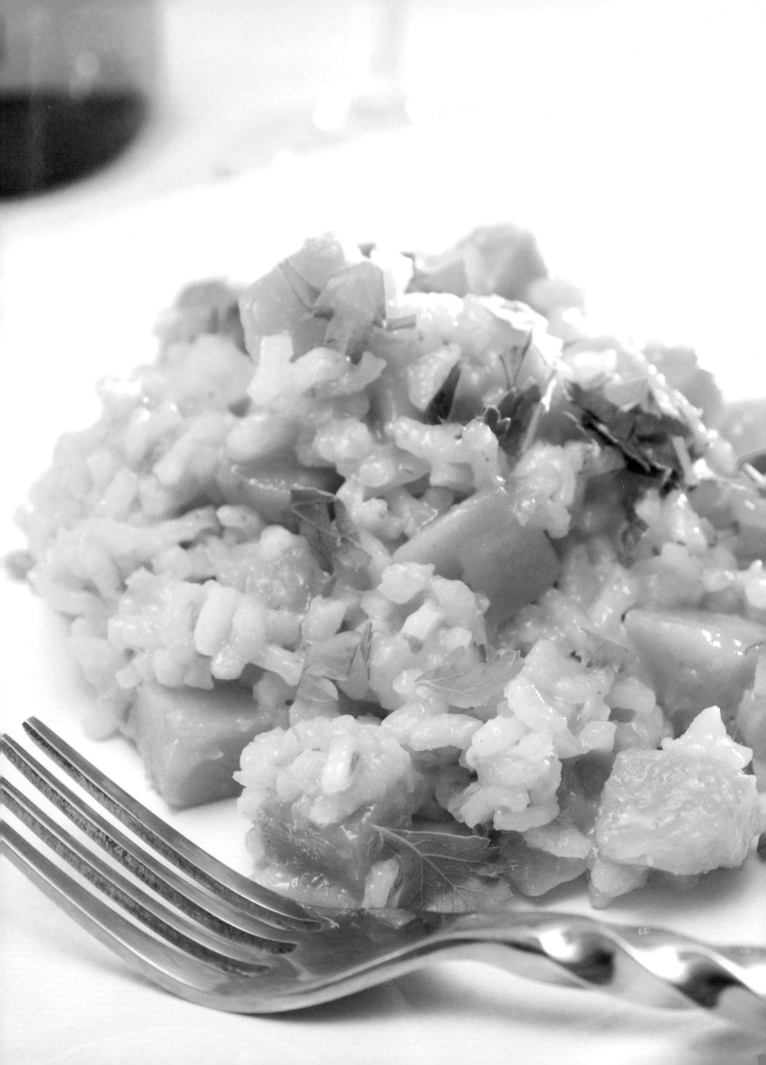

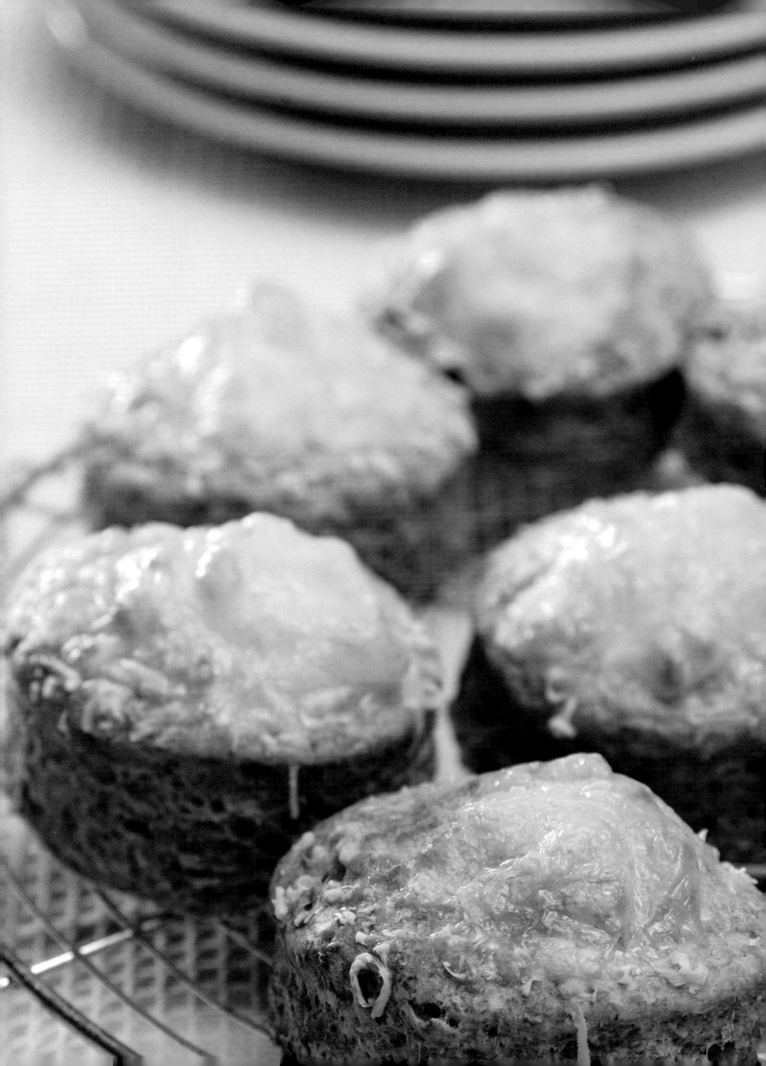

what is diabetes?

Diabetes is having too much sugar (glucose) in your blood. There is no cure and there is no such thing as mild diabetes.

Glucose comes mainly from the digestion of starchy foods such as bread and potatoes, and from sugar, sweets and cakes. The rate at which these foods release glucose in the bloodstream varies: sugary sweet foods give a quicker release of glucose; starchy foods are slower.

We all need glucose as it gives us energy for life. The hormone insulin helps the glucose enter the body's cells where it is converted into energy. If there is too little insulin, or if the insulin does not work properly, the glucose builds up in the bloodstream and causes the classic symptoms of diabetes:

- thirst and a dry mouth
- tiredness
- the need to pass water a lot, especially at night
- loss of weight
- genital itchiness
- blurred vision.

If too much glucose is allowed to build up in the bloodstream it can lead to long-term complications such as

- heart disease
- nerve damage
- kidney disease
- visual impairment.

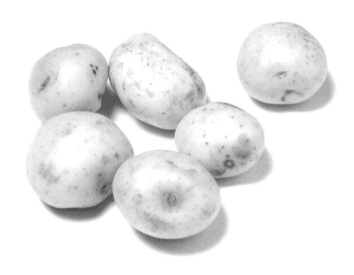

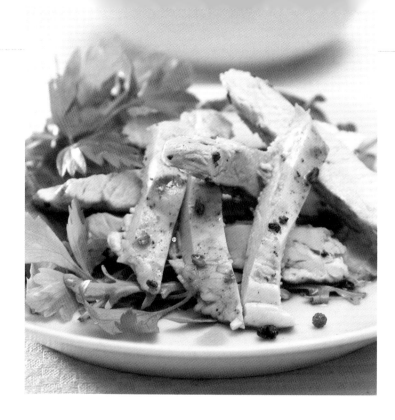

Type I diabetes (insulin-dependent diabetes)

There are two forms of diabetes, Type I and Type II. People with Type I diabetes have a severe shortage of insulin. This needs to be treated with regular injections of insulin and a healthy eating routine. It usually occurs in people under 40.

Type II diabetes (or non insulin-dependent diabetes)

Type II is the most common form of diabetes and accounts for 75% of people with the disease. The body makes some insulin but not enough. This form of diabetes is generally treated by a controlled diet and sometimes additional medication. Most people with Type II diabetes are overweight and over 40 years of age, however with the increase of obesity, increasing numbers of people are being diagnosed with Type II diabetes at an earlier age, and sadly there is an increase in Type II diabetes in children, too.

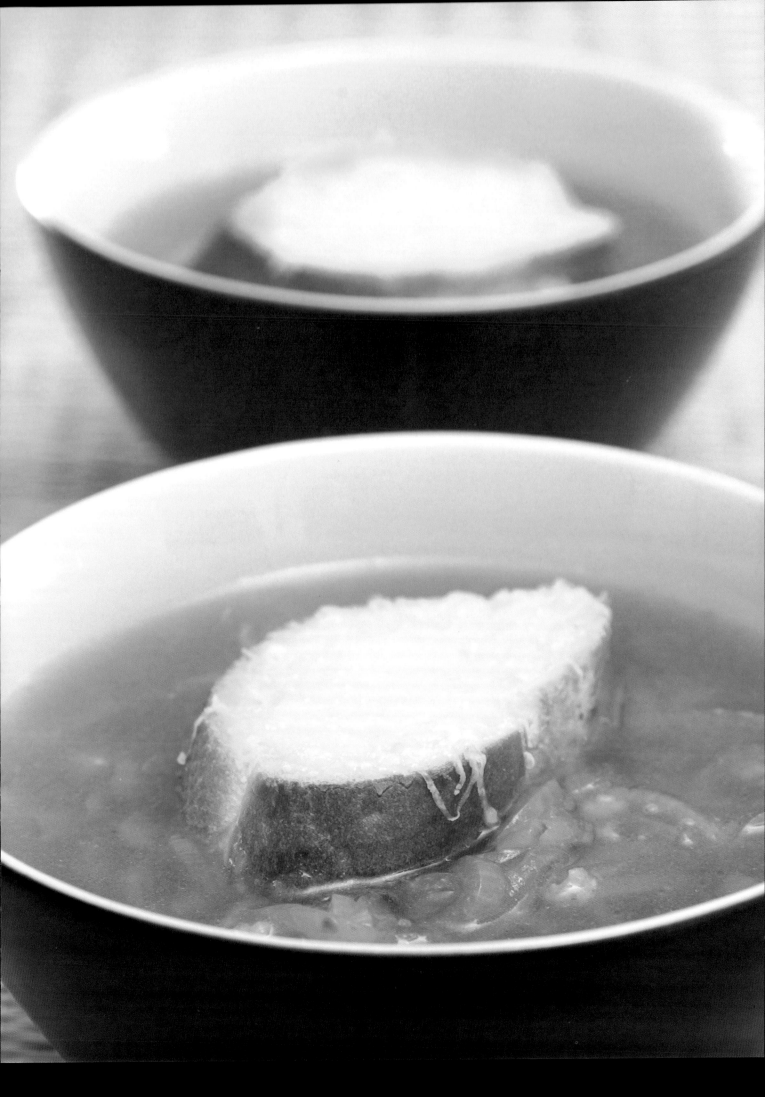

Diet and its role in managing diabetes

Diet plays an integral role in the management and treatment of both types of diabetes, because what, how much and how often you eat can have a significant effect on blood glucose. By making changes to your diet, it is possible to maintain blood sugar levels that are neither too high nor too low. A healthy diet is the key to living with diabetes and to long-term health.

A balanced diet is not only about restricting or excluding foods, it is about balance. There are a few rules to follow:

- eat regular meals
- eat meals that are low in fat especially saturated fat
- eat foods that are low in sugar
- base meals around carbohydrates, not protein or fat
- eat at least five portions of fresh fruit and vegetables per day
- eat a diet that is high in fibre
- add little or no salt
- include oily fish
- have a low alcohol intake
- drinks lots of water
- exercise regularly.

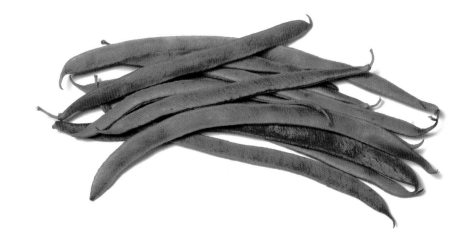

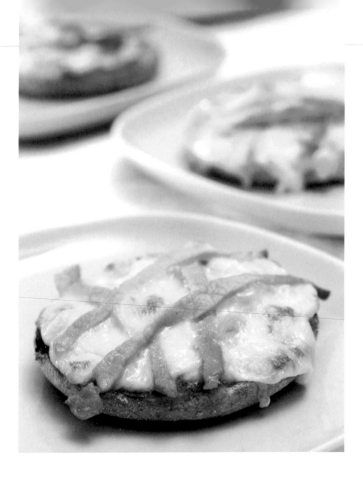

Living with diabetes does not mean you always have to miss out – a few simple changes to lifestyle and eating can make all the difference. However, remember that weight loss can help to control blood glucose levels. If you are overweight, try to eat less and exercise more. Even small adjustments will help, for example eating one snack fewer a day and taking a brisk 5 to 10 minute walk every day. In particular, try to follow a low-fat diet as controlling fat intake will also help to control diabetes.

Of course, we all have times when we want to celebrate, and for the newly diagnosed diabetic this can be the most daunting of all. A little alcohol is permitted, but do not exceed the government's recommendations for alcohol consumption and never drink on an empty stomach. Try to increase the amount of exercise you take around celebrations or festive periods to help balance out any increase of food intake. But don't miss out altogether – just remember to eat smaller portions.

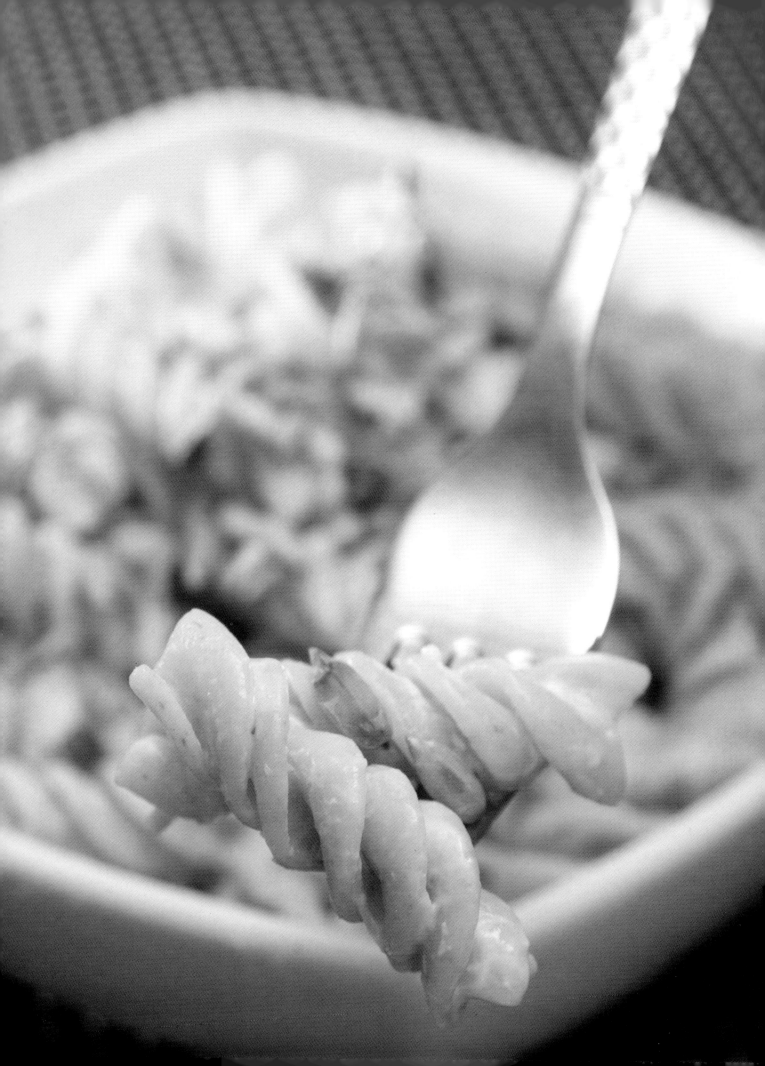

Tips for adopting a healthy diet

Fats and oils

- Use low-fat methods of cooking, such as grilling and baking.
- Use non-stick cookware especially when frying. Cook over a medium-low heat and you will be surprised how little oil is required.
- Reduce the amount of saturated fat by avoiding animal fat as much as possible. Use olive oil instead of butter and cut off visible fat from meat.
- Avoid trans fats from hydrogenated oils and fats (mainly found in processed foods, and usually listed as hydrogenated vegetable oil).
- Use fat-free or low-calorie salad dressing.
- Avoid fast-food outlets as the food tends to be very high in fat and salt.

Carbohydrates

- Complex carbohydrates are made up of simple carbohydrates and fibre. Fibre may be soluble or insoluble. Insoluble fibre has no nutritional value but pushes food through the digestive tract and prevents constipation Soluble fibre slows down the rate at which glucose enters the bloodstream.
- Starchy foods such as bread, pasta, rice and potatoes are naturally low in fat. They are filling so should be used as a basis of all meals.
- Wholegrain foods are higher in fibre, they also convert to glucose more slowly.
- Oats and muesli, sweetcorn, beans and pulses are high in soluble fibre which releases energy even more slowly.
- Serve bread, preferably wholemeal, with meals to increase carbohydrates.

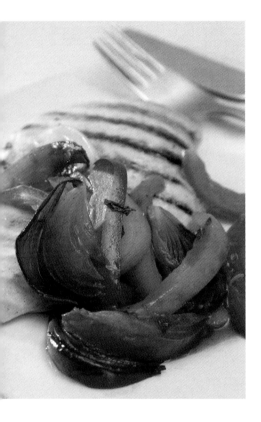

Protein foods

- Meat, fish, nuts, pulses and eggs are rich in protein, minerals and vitamins, but can be high in saturated fat. Use in small amounts at all meals.
- Poultry is a low-fat meat but remember to remove the skin as most of the fat is under it.
- Pulses and beans are both high in soluble fibre and protein and are a good base for a meal.
- Choose lean cuts of meat, for example leg not shoulder, and remove visible fat.
- Use low-fat methods of cooking such as roasting and grilling to cook meat and fish, never deep fry.
- Nuts and seeds are a good source of vitamins and minerals, especially vitamin E and zinc.
- Although oily fish are high in fat they contain omega 3 fatty acids which help prevent heart disease and therefore should be included regularly in the diet.

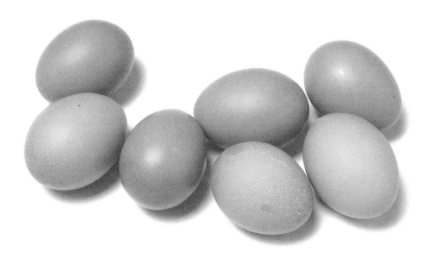

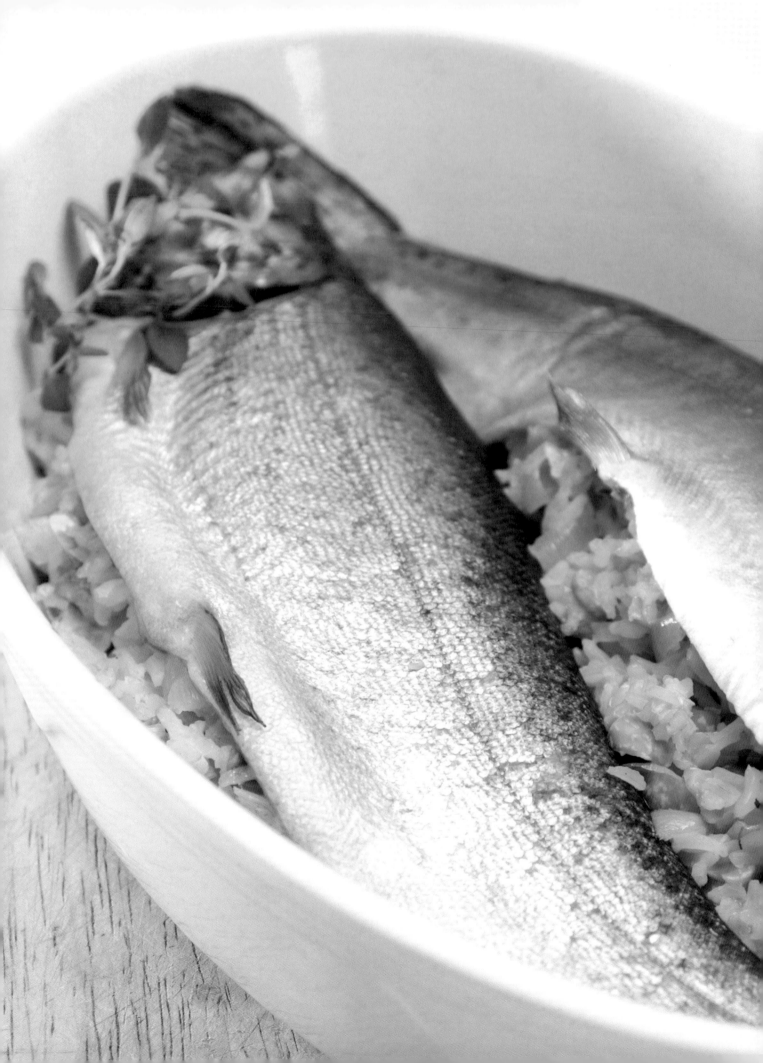

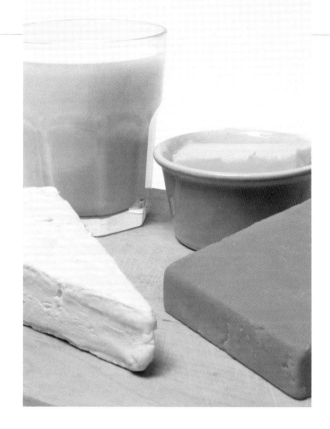

Dairy foods

- Use semi-skimmed or skimmed milk in place of full fat.
- Low-fat fromage frais, reduced-fat Greek-style yoghurt and reduced-fat crème fraîche make good alternatives to cream.
- Some cheeses are high in fat, so check the label. Use cheeses that are naturally lower in fat such as ricotta or feta, or reduced-fat alternatives.

Fruit and vegetables

- Fruit and vegetables are high in fibre, especially soluble fibre.
- Fruit and vegetables contain anti-oxidants which are good for the heart.
- Fruit and vegetables are high in vitamins essential for good health.
- Eat at least five portions of fruit and vegetables a day.
- Sweetcorn is especially high in soluble fibre.
- Remember that frozen vegetables can be as high in vitamins as fresh vegetables.
- Use canned fruit in fruit juice, not syrup.
- Fruit juices can raise blood glucose quickly as the natural fruit sugars in the juice are in a liquid form which is more readily absorbed. Drink fruit juice with a meal and dilute with water.
- Do not add butter to cooked vegetables – avoid altogether or use olive oil instead.

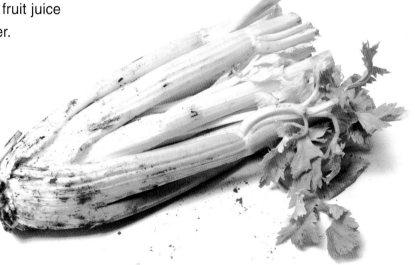

Sugars and sweet foods

- Simple carbohydrates such as sugar are converted to glucose almost immediately and should be limited.
- Small amounts can be eaten with other foods without having too much of a detrimental effect on glucose levels.
- Avoid foods and drinks where sugar is the main ingredient, particularly between meals.
- Eat unsweetened breakfast cereals.

Sweet foods do not have to be cut out completely, even if a food is very sugary. Think about how much and how often you eat that food. For example, although jam has a high sugar content you eat only a little, so the small amount should not adversely effect blood glucose levels.

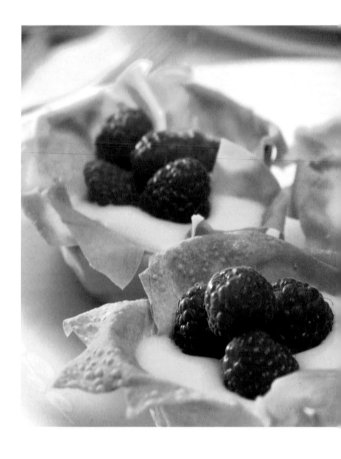

Alcohol

- Keep to safe limits: 21–28 units per week for men, 14–21 units per week for women.
- Have two to three alcohol-free days per week.
- Do not binge drink.
- Never drink alcohol on an empty stomach to avoid low blood sugar.
- Alternate alcoholic drinks with non-alcoholic drinks.

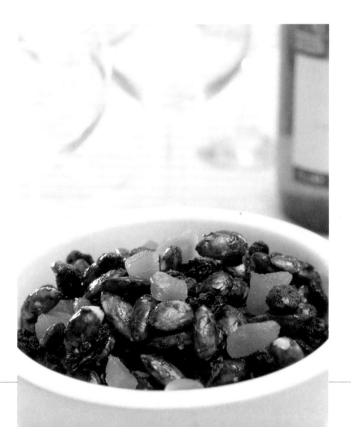

How to use this book to follow a healthy diet

Whether you have been diagnosed as Type I or Type II diabetes, your doctor will advise you in the use of drugs, injections and glucose testing. He or she will almost certainly give you dietary advice or send you to a dietician. Always follow this advice.

The recipes in the book have been written to take account of the current dietary advice for people with diabetes. In fact, this is the healthy diet that we should all be eating, so the recipes will suit people without diabetes as well.

The recipes are all low-sugar and low-fat. Some recipes have serving suggestions to keep within the dietary guidelines, and should be followed whenever possible.

The book has been divided into chapters with meal suggestions throughout the day. You will also find recipes for healthy snacks and drinks as well as some recipes for cakes and desserts which are lower in fat and sugar than traditional recipes, allowing you to include these in the diet occasionally without pushing the guidelines too far.

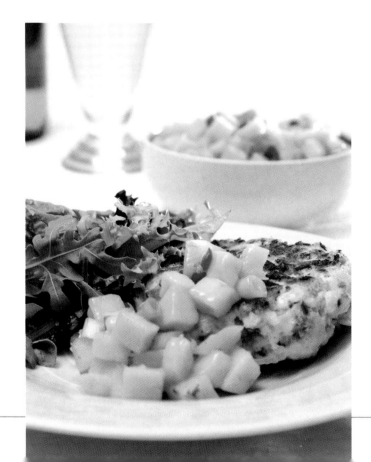

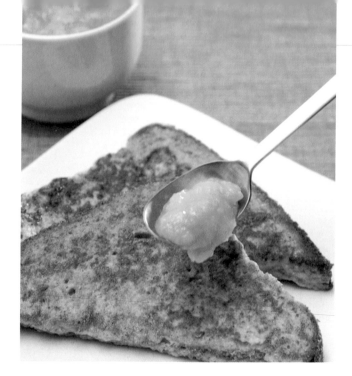

Breakfast

The most important meal of the day, breakfast should never be skipped. Your body has effectively gone through a period of fasting during the night, so blood sugars will be low and should not be allowed to drop any lower.

Avoid high sugar/fat dishes which will release energy too quickly. If choosing a breakfast cereal choose a high-fibre unsweetened cereal, or make your own muesli (see pages 30–3). In addition to the other suggestions in the chapter, you could serve the muffins from the baking chapter (see pages 206–9) or serve a simple cooked breakfast such as poached, scrambled or boiled eggs with wholemeal toast, or tomatoes on toast with a lean back rasher of bacon.

Lunch

It is vital to eat regular meals, so lunch is also important. Do not skip lunch even if you are trying to lose weight. Your blood sugars will drop during the afternoon and you may be tempted to reach for a less healthy snack to make up for it.

There are plenty of lunch ideas in this chapter, both hot and cold. There are some suitable for those who need a packed lunch. You can also serve meals consisting of a small portion of fish or meat, plus a vegetable or a salad for lunch. But remember the importance of including some carbohydrate such as rice, potatoes or bread as this will release energy slowly over the afternoon.

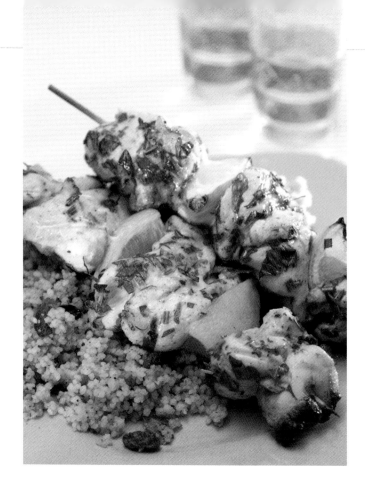

Dinner

The main meals featured in this chapter are based around carbohydrate, or have a serving suggestion that adds the required carbohydrates. There is a recipe suitable for all occasions. If you prefer to eat your main meal at midday, simply serve the dinner recipes at midday and serve the lunch suggestions in the evenings.

Desserts and bakes

Both cakes and desserts can be enjoyed in small quantities. It is important to eat five portions of fruit and vegetables a day, so a fruit dessert can help you to achieve this. The cakes and bakes have been adapted to reduce the fat and sugar content. Nevertheless, it is important to remember that most cakes and desserts should be eaten only as occasional treats.

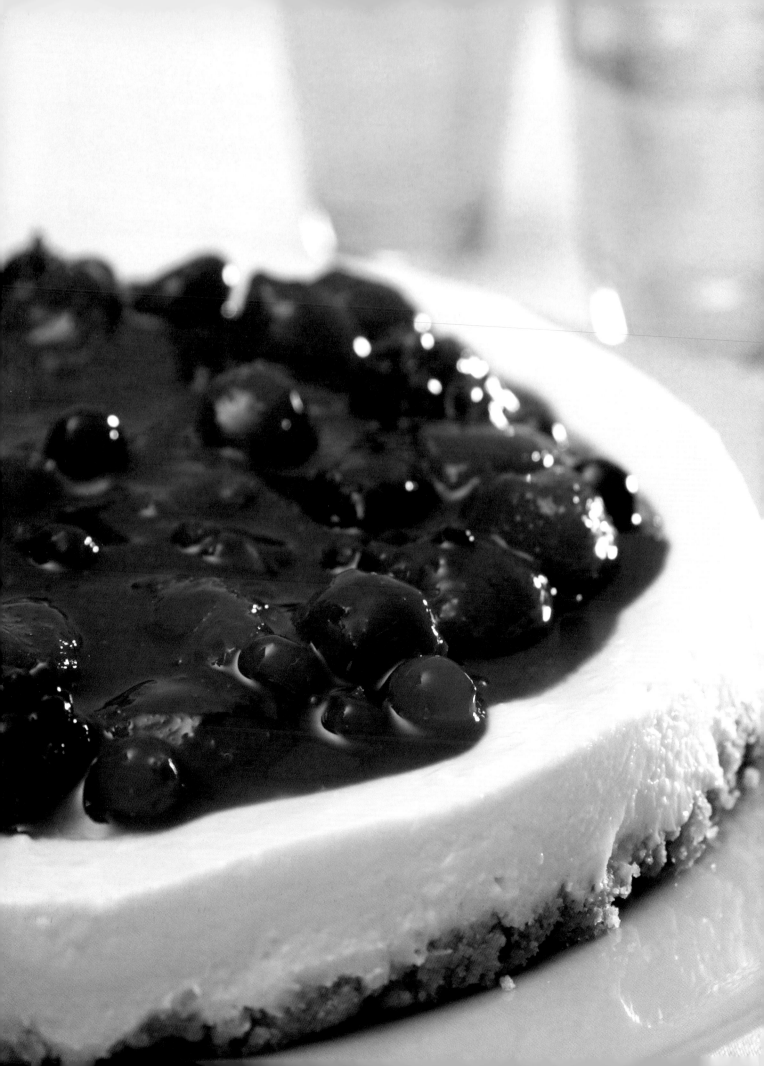

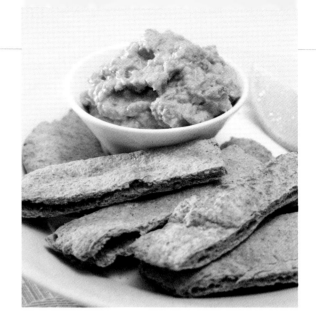

Snacks

It is important that people with diabetes do not overload their bodies with food, and that they eat regular moderate-sized meals with two to three small snacks in between. This will help to keep blood sugar levels steady during the day, avoiding highs and lows. You will find ideas for healthy savoury snacks, many of which can be prepared in advance to be nibbled over a couple of days. Moderation remains the key here. If you prefer a sweet snack you can try one of the many delicious low-fat, low-sugar bakes in the desserts and bakes chapter. But again remember – moderation. A reduced-sugar cake will not be low-sugar if you eat two large slices! Don't forget, you can also snack on fruit, low-fat yoghurt and raw vegetables.

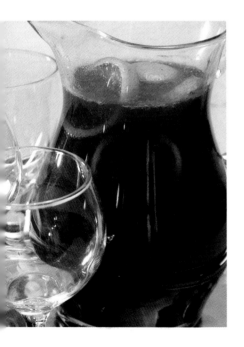

Drinks

Also included are some ideas for healthy drinks. Fizzy, sugary drinks are out and you may prefer to limit your intake of artificial sweetener. Here you will find alternatives, many of which are ideal when entertaining as well as for enjoying at home.

If you want to be in control of your diet, eat well and easily, then this book is for you.

Enjoy!

Tips for Successful Cooking

- Use metric or imperial measurements only; do not mix the two.

- Use measuring spoons: 1 tsp = 5ml; 1 tbsp = 15ml

- All spoon measurements are level unless otherwise stated.

- All eggs are medium unless otherwise stated.

- Recipes using raw or lightly cooked eggs should not be given to babies, pregnant women, the very old or anyone suffering from or recovering from an illness.

- The cooking times are an approximate guide only. If you are using a fan oven reduce the cooking time according to the manufacturer's instructions.

- Ovens should be preheated to the required temperature.

- Fruits and vegetables should be washed before use.

Please note – most of the recipes have ingredients listed for a number of servings. If the recipe includes servings for two and four people, for example, the recipe will show how much to add for two people, with the amount for four people in brackets. e.g.: 2 tbsp (4 tbsp).

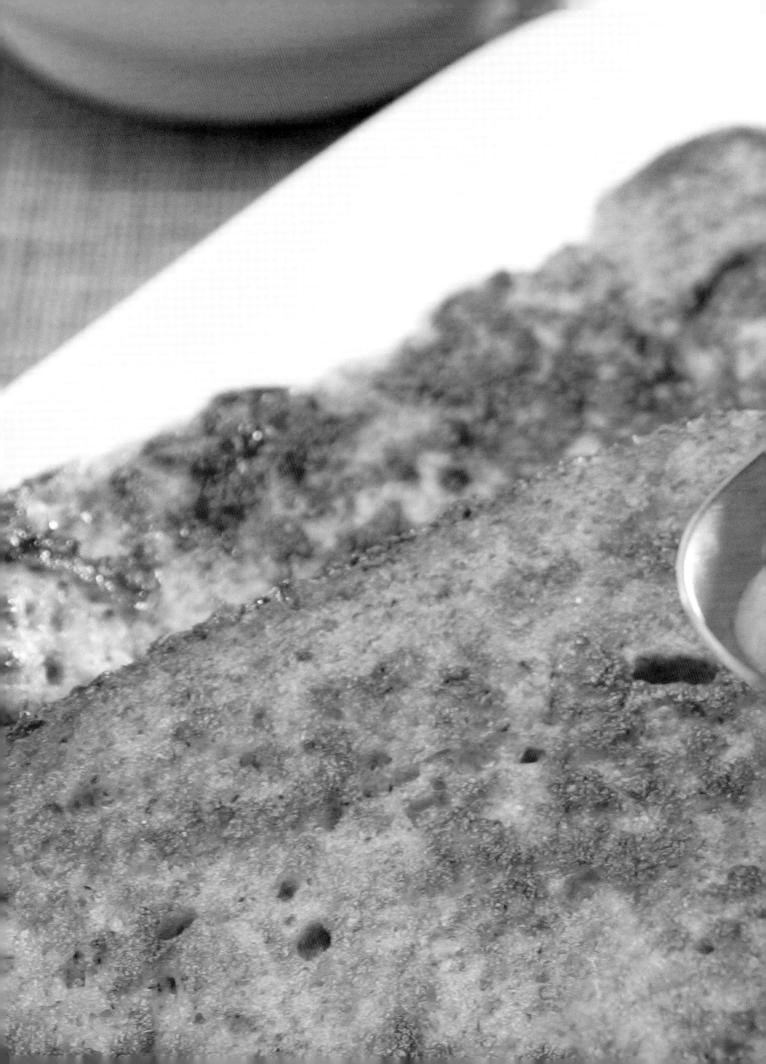

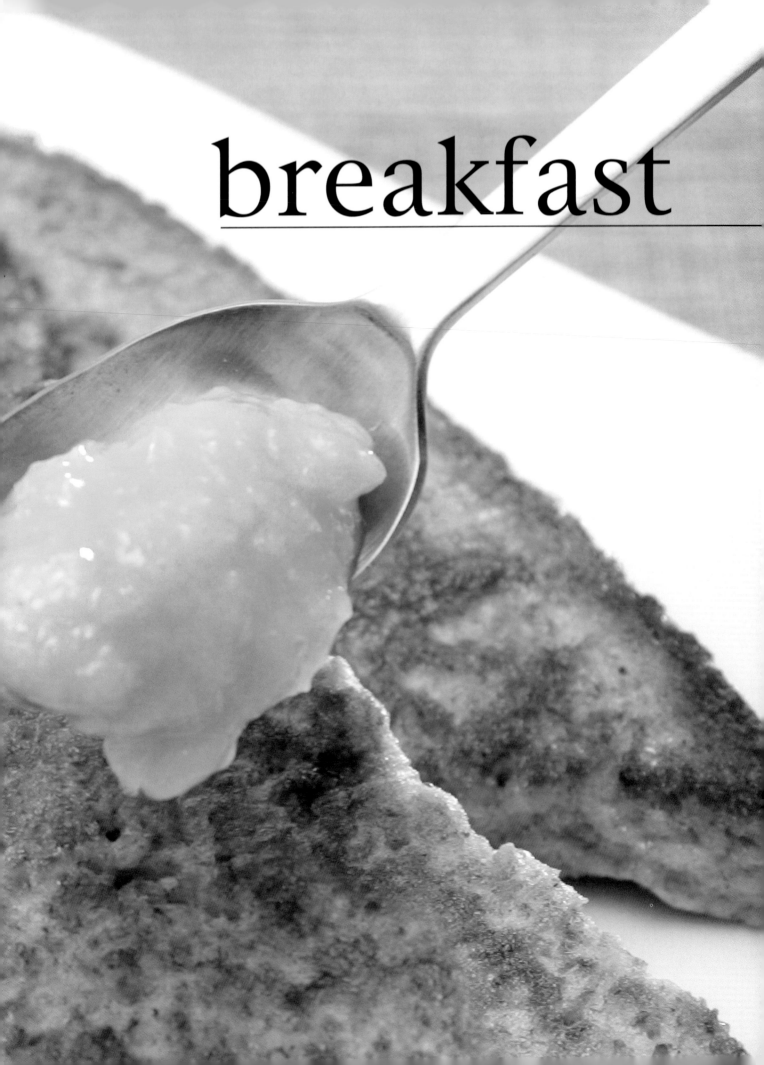

breakfast

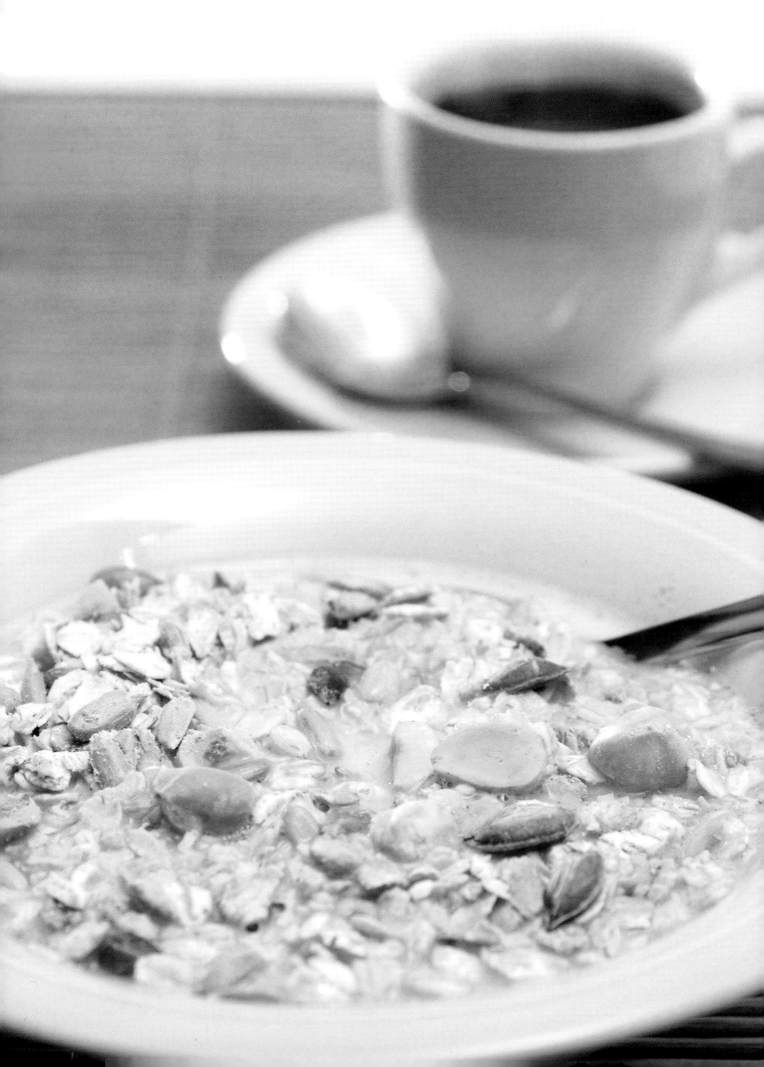

Seedy Home-made Muesli

Quick and Easy

Muesli is an ideal breakfast as it has plenty of soluble fibre for a slow release of energy throughout the morning. This mix is full of seeds which have lots of trace elements and minerals essential for good health. You can also add some dried fruit if you prefer. Try not to add too much sugar – instead try sweetening with date syrup which is full of natural sweetness.

Makes 400g/14oz (enough for 8 servings)

25g/1oz hazel nuts
4 tbsp sunflower seeds
4 tbsp pumpkin seeds
1 tbsp sesame seeds
225g/8oz rolled oats
50g/2oz wheat flakes
50g/2oz barley flakes
1 tsp mixed spice

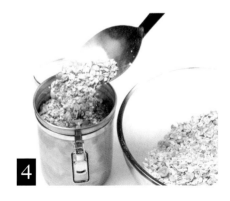

1 Toast the hazelnuts until golden. Roughly chop.

2 Toast the seeds.

3 Mix all the ingredients together.

4 Store in an airtight container.

5 Serve with a low-fat natural yoghurt, skimmed or semi-skimmed milk, or unsweetened fruit juice.

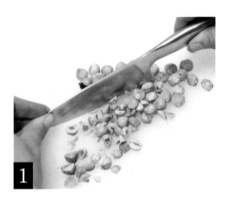

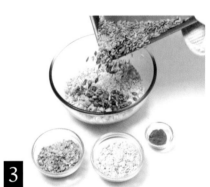

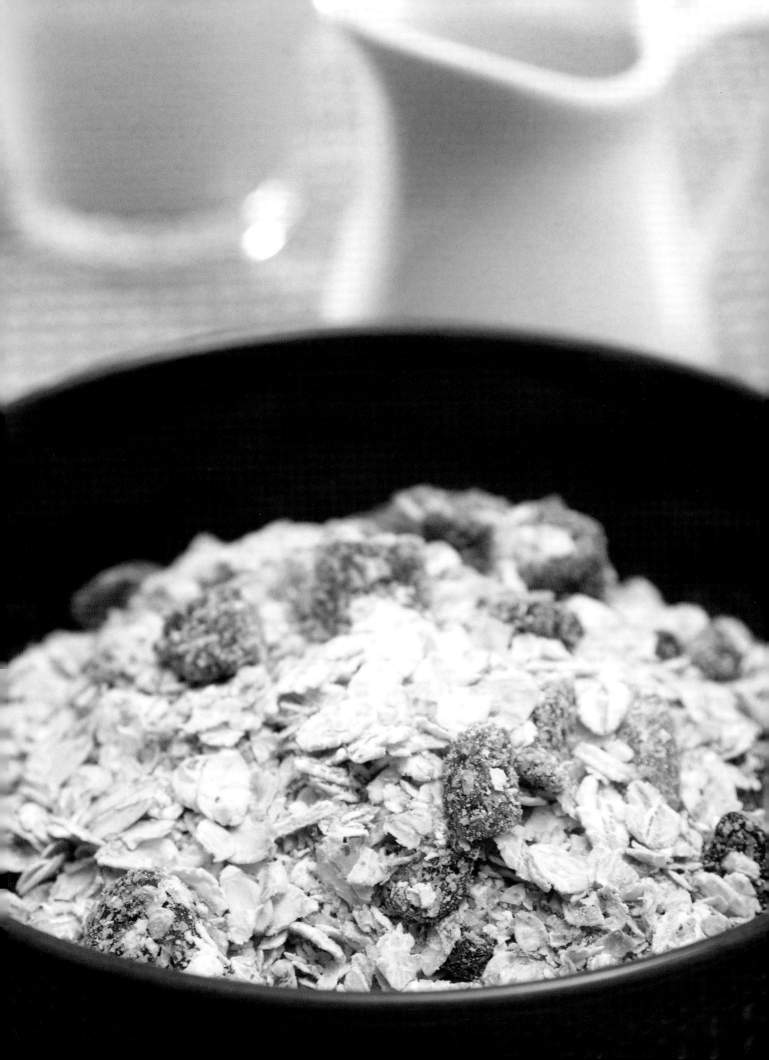

Home-made Muesli with Dried Fruit

Prepare Ahead

This is a traditional-style muesli with lots of dried fruit. It is sweet, so you should be able to avoid adding extra sugar. While you can buy ready-made unsweetened muesli, the great thing about making your own is that you can vary it to your own taste, so feel free to play around with the proportions of the ingredients until you have your favourite blend.

Makes 600g/1lb 5oz (enough for 12 servings)

50g/2oz no-soak dried figs
50g/2oz no-soak dried apricots
50g/2oz dried dates
175g/6oz rolled oats
50g/2oz rye flakes
50g/2oz wheat germ
50g/2oz sultanas

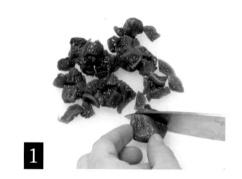

1 Chop the figs, apricots and dates.

2 Mix all the ingredients together and store in an airtight container.

3 Serve with low-fat natural yoghurt, skimmed or semi-skimmed milk, or unsweetened fruit juice.

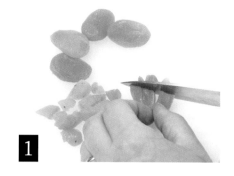

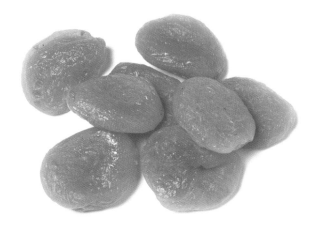

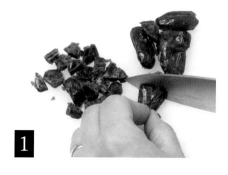

Porridge with Apple Purée

Family Favourite

I used to like my porridge sweetened with lots of sugar until I discovered how good it could taste with a fruit purée stirred in, rather like adding jam to rice pudding. Porridge made with oatmeal has the best texture and is the slowest to release energy to the body, helping to keep blood glucose levels even. Rolled oats can also be used, and they will cook in about half the time. Instant oat porridge, which is very finely ground, is converted quickly to glucose in the body, so should not be eaten by people with diabetes.

Ingredients for 1

225ml/8fl oz water
75ml/2½fl oz skimmed or
  semi-skimmed milk
25g/1oz medium oatmeal
½-1 tsp golden caster sugar
pinch of salt

Apple purée

1 large green eating apple
2 tbsp water
1 tbsp barley malt syrup
¼ tsp ground cinnamon

Ingredients for 2

450ml/¾pt water
150ml/¼pt skimmed or semi-
  skimmed milk
50g/2oz medium oatmeal
1-2 tsp golden caster sugar
¼ tsp salt

Apple purée:

2 large green eating apples
4 tbsp water
2 tbsp barley malt syrup
½ tsp ground cinnamon

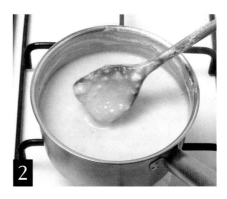

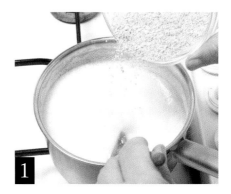

1 Bring the water and milk to a boil in a saucepan and slowly stir in the oatmeal. Add the sugar if using and salt.

2 Simmer gently for 20 minutes, stirring occasionally to begin with and more constantly towards the end of the cooking time to prevent it from sticking to the base of the pan.

3 Meanwhile peel, core and slice the apples and place in a small pan with the water, malt syrup and cinnamon.

4 Cook over a medium heat, breaking up the apple with the side of a spoon as it softens and cooks. Beat to a chunky purée.

5 Serve the porridge with the apple purée spooned on top.

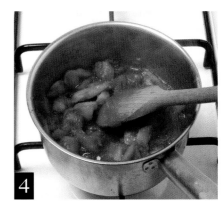

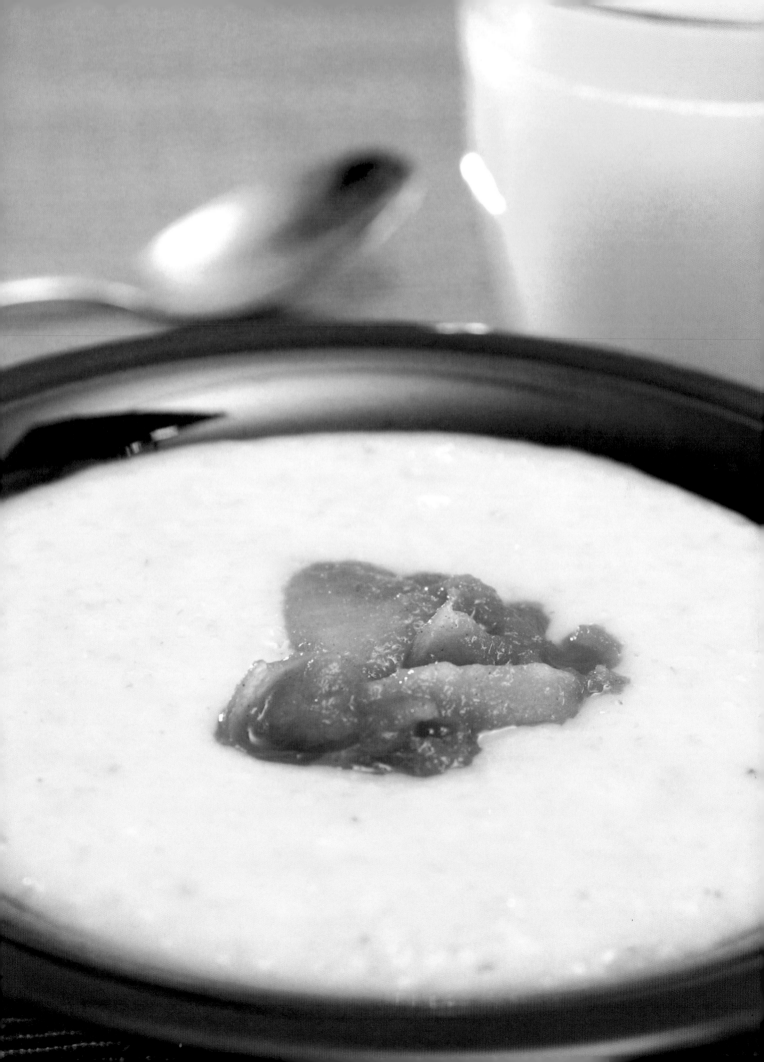

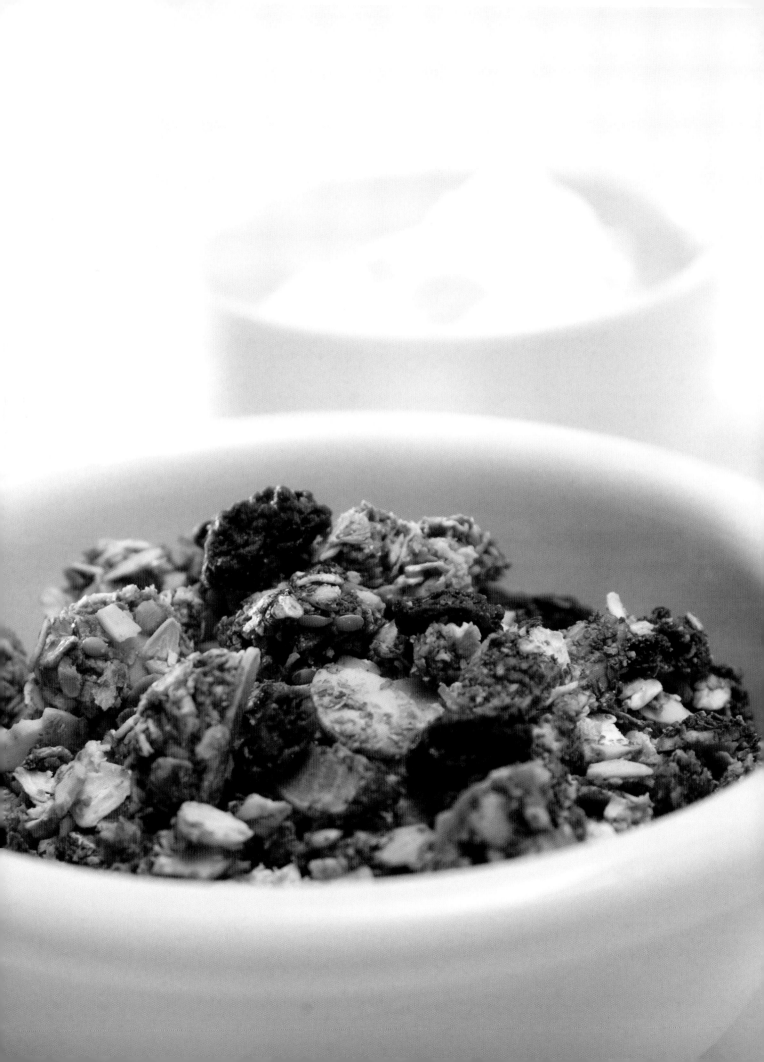

Granola

Prepare Ahead

This is an American crunchy breakfast cereal which is very easy to make at home. Serve with milk or yoghurt. Granola is also delicious as a nibble at any time of the day. Barley malt syrup can be bought in health food shops and is a delicious alternative to sugar and honey. Honey could also be used as an alternative in this recipe.

Makes about 450g/1lb (enough for 8 servings)

225g/8oz rolled oats
75g/3oz wheatgerm
75g/3oz flaked almonds
1 tbsp sunflower seeds or linseeds
½ tsp ground cinnamon or freshly grated nutmeg
3 tbsp barley malt syrup
1 tbsp boiling water
2 tbsp sunflower oil
1 tsp vanilla essence
75g/3oz raisins

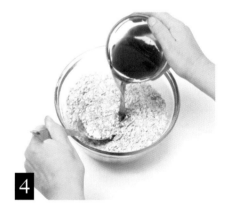

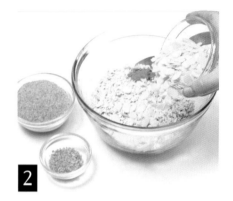

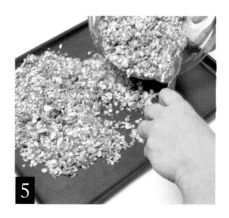

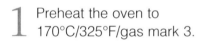

1 Preheat the oven to 170°C/325°F/gas mark 3.

2 Mix together the oats, wheatgerm, almonds, seeds and cinnamon or nutmeg.

3 Place the barley malt syrup in a small bowl and stir in the boiling water.

4 Stir in the oil and vanilla essence. Drizzle over the oat mixture and stir until the oats are well coated.

5 Spread out in a shallow roasting tin and bake for 25–30 minutes until golden, stirring once or twice.

6 Stir in the raisins.

7 Leave to cool then break up into chunks. Store in an airtight container in a cool place for up to 1 month.

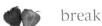
Yogurt with Berry Compote

This is a delicious light breakfast, and although berries are cheapest in the summer it can also be made with frozen fruit, so it is suitable for all year round.

Ingredients for 1

**125g/4½oz mixed summer
   berries, e.g. strawberries,
   blackberries, raspberries,
   red and black currants
2 tbsp orange juice
1-2 tsp clear honey
1 tsp cornflour
150g/5oz reduced-fat Greek-
   style yoghurt**

Ingredients for 2

**250g/9oz mixed summer
   berries, e.g. strawberries,
   blackberries, raspberries,
   red and black currants
4 tbsp orange juice
1 tbsp clear honey
2 tsp cornflour
300g/10½oz reduced-fat
   Greek-style yoghurt**

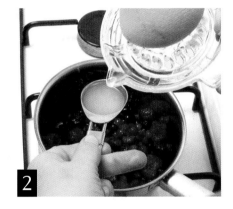

1 Wash and hull the berries if required. Shake off excess water.

2 Place in a small pan with the orange juice and honey.

3 Cook gently until the juices begin to run.

4 Mix the cornflour with 1 tbsp (2tbsp) water and stir into the pan. Heat gently stirring until sauce thickens.

5 Allow to cool covered with a piece of wetted greaseproof paper (this prevents a skin forming). Chill until required.

6 Serve the berry compote with the yoghurt.

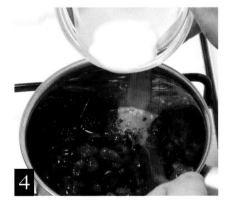

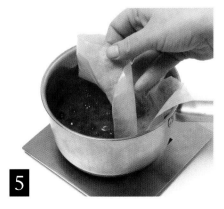

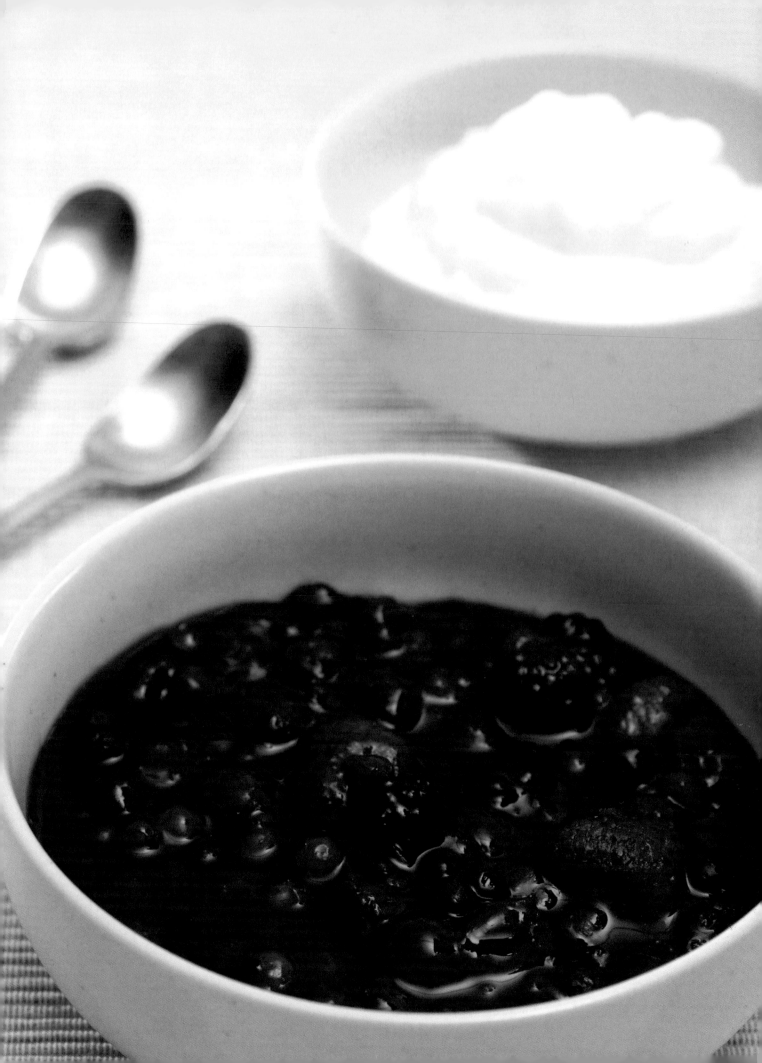

Citrus Fruit Salad

Quick and Easy

As with the other fruit-based breakfasts, this will count towards your 5 portions of fruit and vegetables a day. It is a good idea to include some carbohydrate too, so serve some wholemeal toast or a plain wholemeal biscuit or muffin.

Ingredients for 2

1 grapefruit
1 orange
2 tsp clear honey
1 tbsp lemon juice
½ tsp chopped fresh mint

Ingredients for 4

2 grapefruits
2 oranges
4 tsp clear honey
2 tbsp lemon juice
1 tsp chopped fresh mint

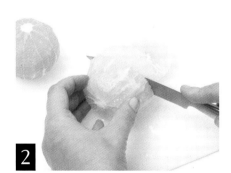

1 Using a sharp knife, cut the peel and pith away from the grapefruit and orange.

2 Slice thinly. Arrange on small individual plates. Keep cool until required

3 Whisk together the honey and lemon juice and drizzle over the sliced fruit.

4 Sprinkle over the chopped mint and serve.

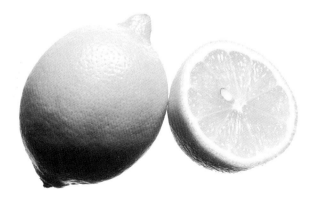

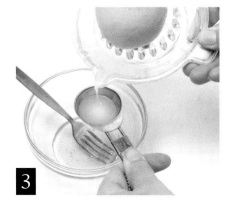

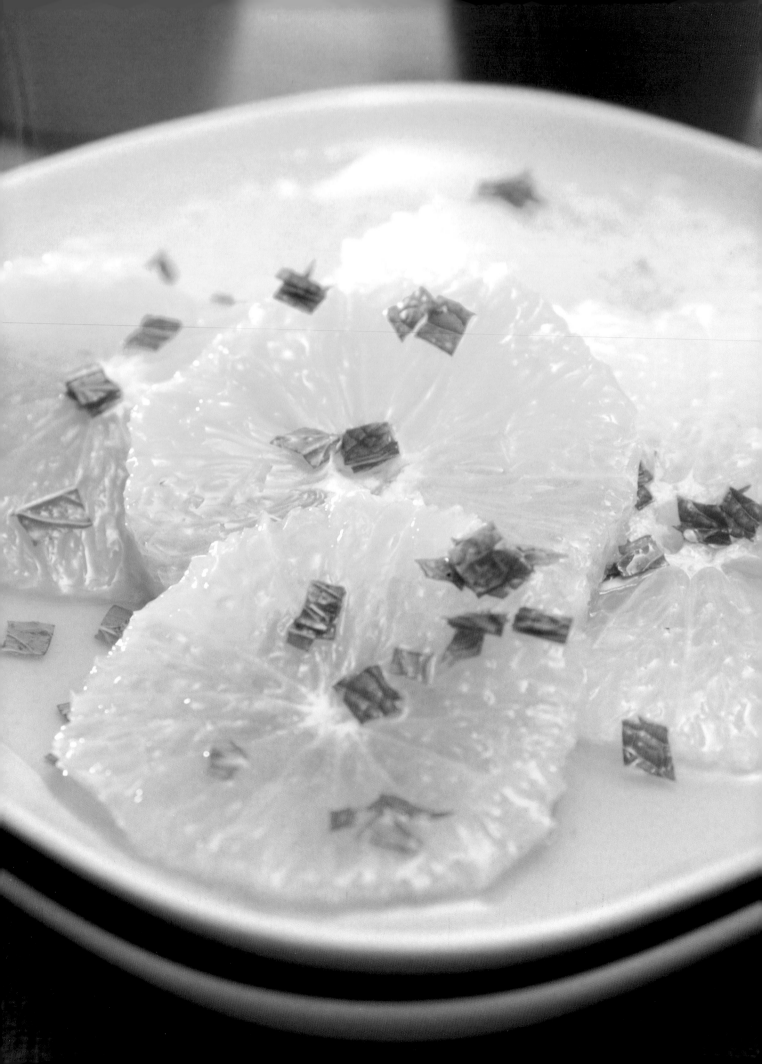

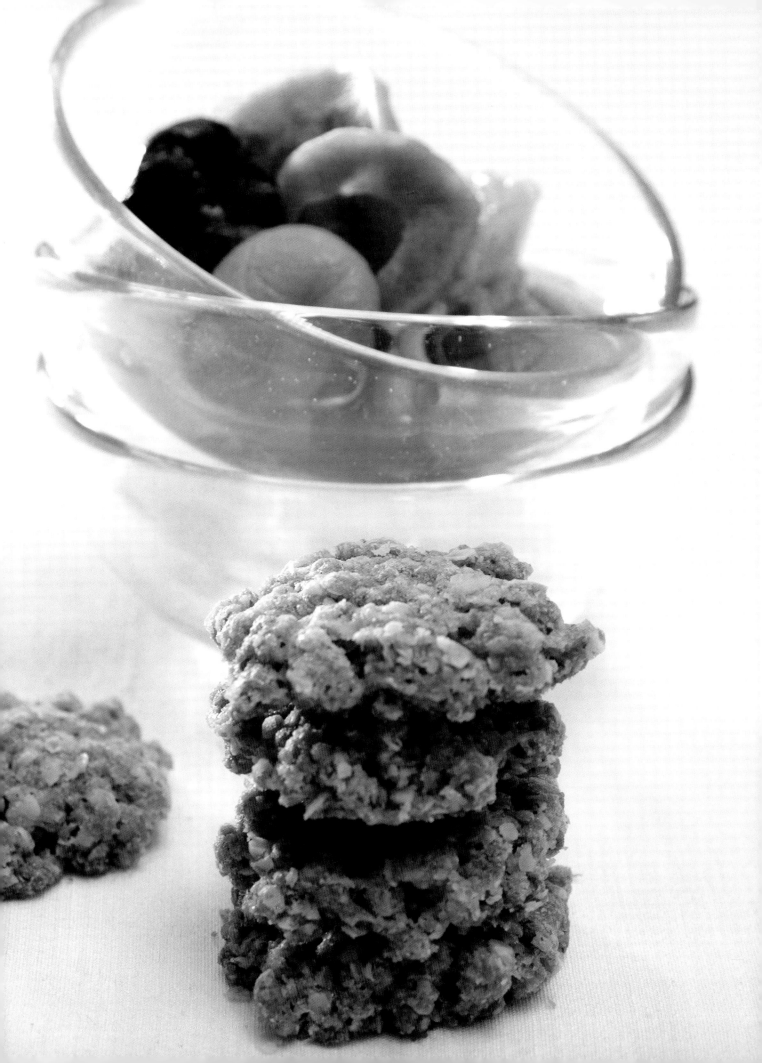

Dried Fruit Compote with Wholemeal Biscuits

This is a great fruit breakfast that is available all year round. The biscuits add carbohydrate to the meal. You can buy bags of mixed dried fruit salad, or alternatively buy a selection of your favourite dried fruits. Dried fruits are great for nibbling on during the day if you feel peckish. Both the compote and the biscuits can be made in advance. Allow 2 biscuits per person for breakfast, the remaining biscuits can be stored in an airtight tin for up to 1 week.

Ingredients for 2

Dried fruit compote:

75ml/2½fl oz water
150ml/¼pt unsweetened apple juice
150g/5oz dried fruit salad
pinch of mixed spice

Ingredients for 4

Dried fruit compote:

150ml/¼pt water
300ml/½pt unsweetened apple juice
275g/10oz dried fruit salad
¼ tsp mixed spice

Biscuits (makes about 18):

100g/4oz rolled oats
100g/4oz plain wholemeal flour
75g/3oz light muscovado sugar
150ml/5fl oz sunflower oil
1 egg
1 tsp mixed spice

1 To make the fruit compote, place all the ingredients in a saucepan and bring slowly to the boil.

2 Reduce the heat, cover and simmer gently for 40 minutes until the fruit is just tender. Allow to cool and chill until required.

3 To make the biscuits, preheat the oven to 180°C/350°F/gas mark 4.

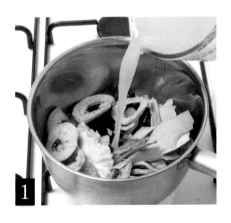

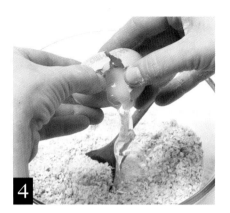

4 Place all the ingredients for the biscuits in a large mixing bowl and beat until they are well combined.

5 Take a small amount of the mixture and press together to form a ball about the size of a walnut. Place on lightly greased baking trays. Flatten slightly.

6 Bake for 10–15 minutes until golden. Allow to cool on the baking tray for a few minutes before transferring to a wire rack to cool completely.

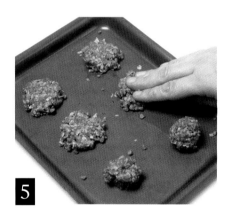

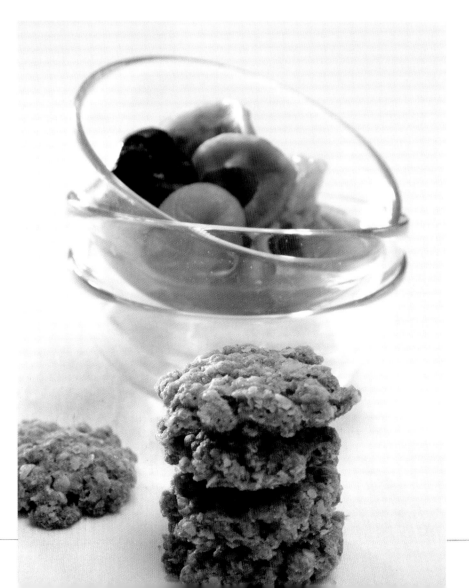

Drop Pancakes with Orange & Strawberries

The pancakes can be made in advance and reheated in a warm oven, or for a few seconds in the microwave. They can also be frozen. The orange and strawberries can be prepared the night before and left overnight in the refrigerator.

Ingredients for 2

1 orange, peeled and
    segmented
75g/3oz strawberries,
    washed and hulled
1 tbsp orange juice

Pancakes:

50g/2oz plain flour
15g/½oz golden caster sugar
½ tsp baking powder
75ml/2½fl oz low-fat natural
    yoghurt
1 egg
a little sunflower oil

Ingredients for 4

2 oranges, peeled and
    segmented
175g/6oz strawberries,
    washed and hulled
2 tbsp orange juice

Pancakes:

100g/4oz plain flour
25g/1oz golden caster sugar
1 tsp baking powder
150ml/¼pt low-fat natural
    yoghurt
2 eggs
a little sunflower oil

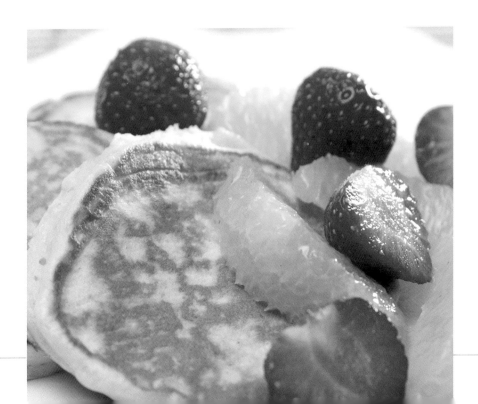

1 Place the oranges and strawberries, halved or quartered if desired, in a small bowl and pour over the orange juice. Cover and chill until required.

2 To make the pancakes, sift the flour into a bowl and stir in the sugar and baking powder.

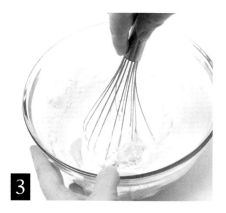

3 Add the yoghurt and eggs and beat until smooth.

4 Heat a heavy-based non-stick frying pan or flat griddle pan and lightly oil.

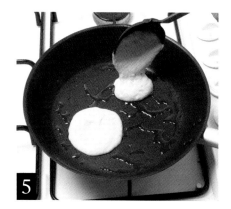

5 Drop a large tablespoon of the batter mixture into the pan and spread slightly. Repeat with one or two more spoonfuls, depending on the size of the pan, to make several small pancakes.

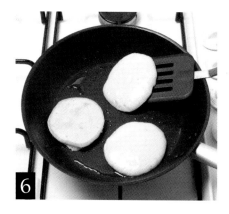

6 Cook for about 2 minutes until golden on the underside. Flip over and cook for another 1–2 minutes.

7 Remove from the pan and keep warm. Repeat with the remaining mixture.

8 Serve the pancakes with the orange and strawberries.

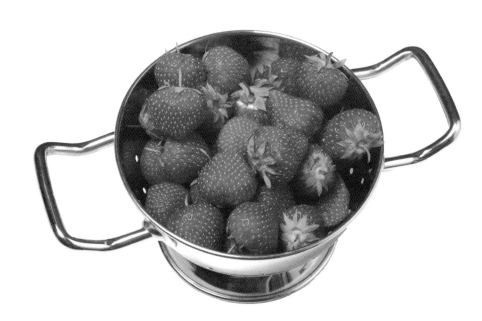

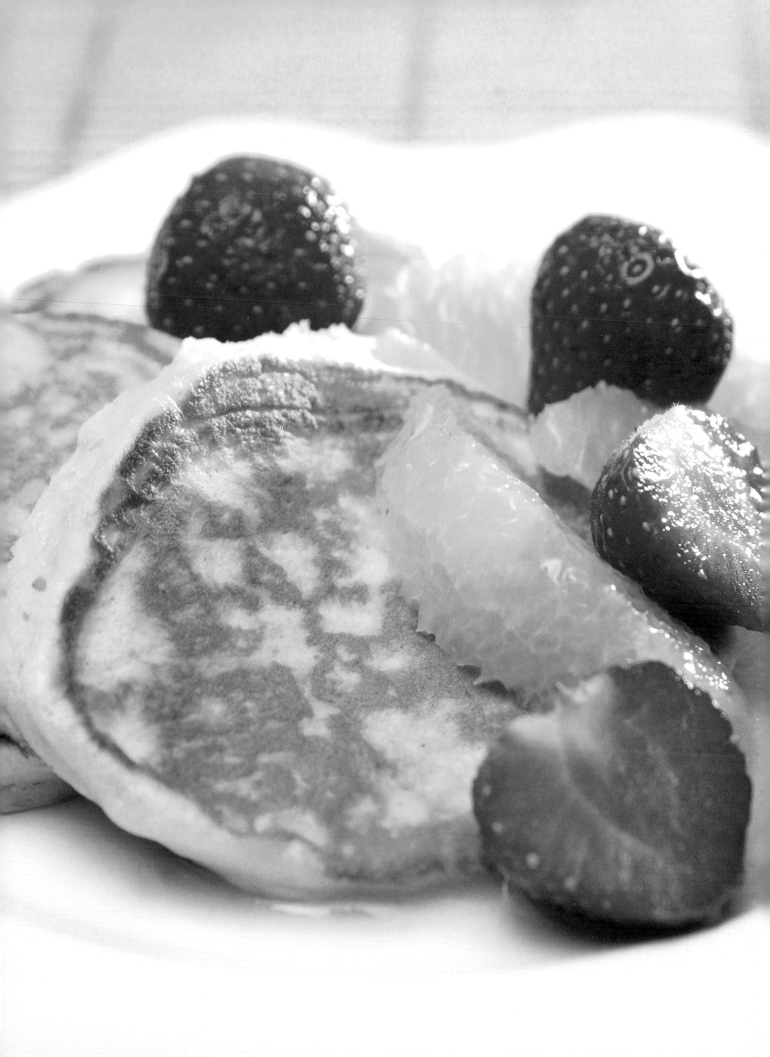

French Toast with Apricot Sauce

It is hard to cut down the quantities for this breakfast treat, so I tend to serve it at the weekends when we all sit down for breakfast together. The apricot sauce can be made the night before and can be served hot or cold. If you use a non-stick pan you will need very little oil to cook the toasts.

Ingredients for 4

Apricot sauce:

100g/4oz no-soak dried apricots, chopped
150ml/¼pt orange juice
150ml/¼pt water
¼ tsp freshly grated nutmeg

French toast:

1 large egg
100ml/3½fl oz skimmed or semi-skimmed milk
generous pinch of freshly grated nutmeg
4 slices bread, preferably wholemeal
a little sunflower oil

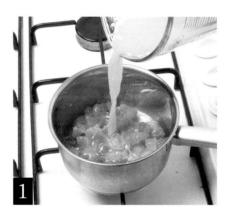

1 To make the apricot sauce, place all the ingredients in a small saucepan and bring slowly to the boil.

2 Reduce the heat, cover and simmer gently for 15 minutes. Purée in a food processor or liquidiser. Keep warm or chill if required.

3 To make the toasts, lightly beat the egg to break it up, then beat in the milk and nutmeg.

4 Cut the bread slices in half. Dip the bread in the beaten egg mixture until it is well coated.

5 Heat the oil in a heavy-based non-stick frying pan and cook the bread for 1–2 minutes on each side until golden. You will need to do this in batches. Keep warm. Serve with the apricot sauce.

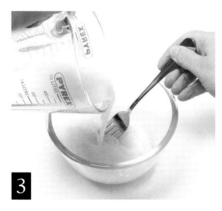

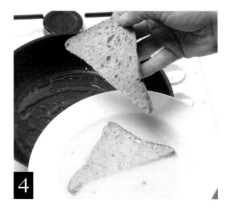

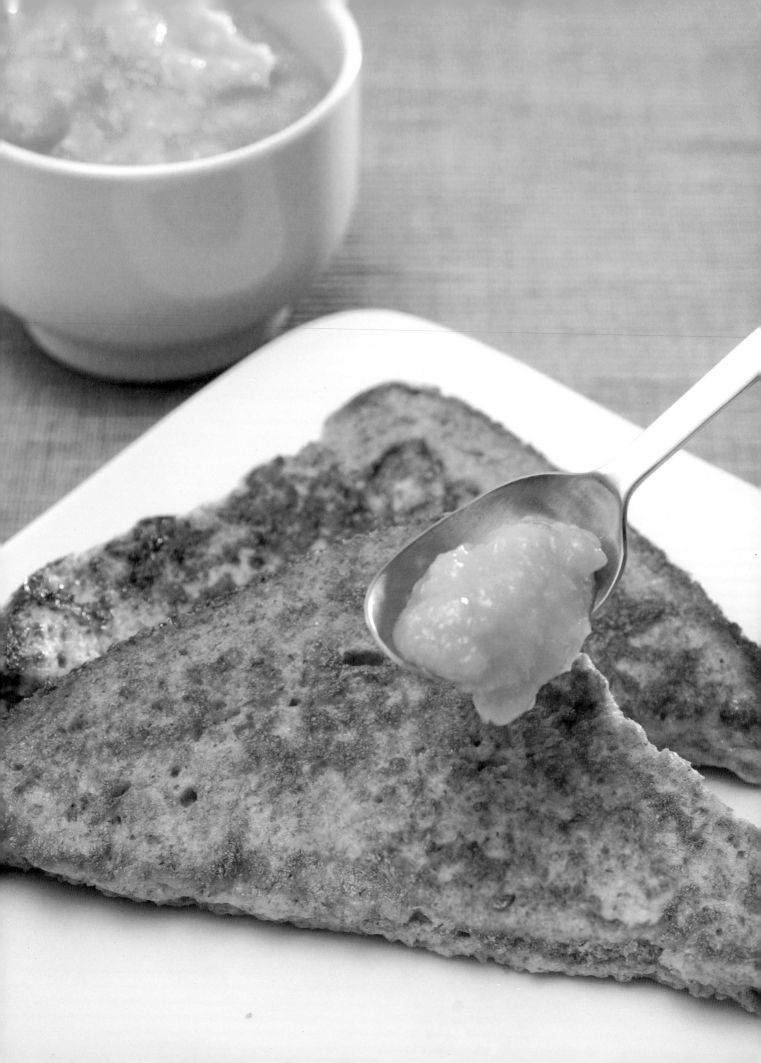

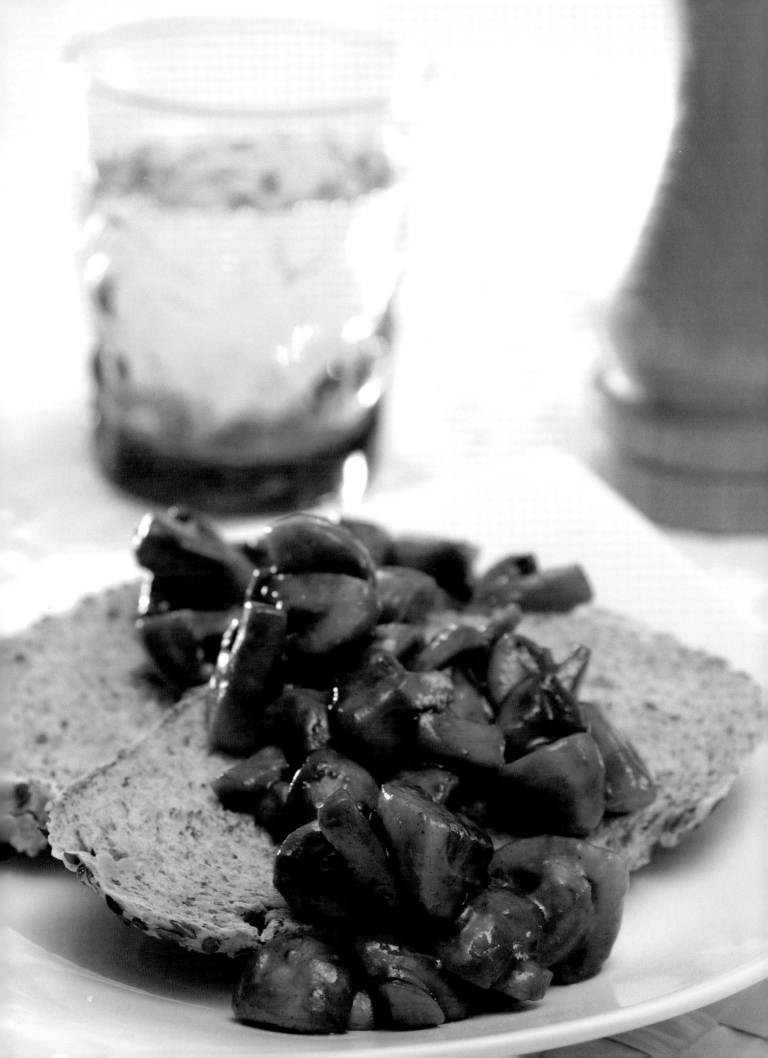

Savoury Mushroom Toast

Quick and Easy

For those who prefer a savoury breakfast this is a good choice. It is simple to make, has loads of flavour and the mushrooms count towards your daily five portions of fruit and vegetables.

Ingredients for 1

1 tsp olive oil
75g/3oz button mushrooms,
    quartered
1 tsp brown fruity sauce
1 tsp tomato ketchup
½ tsp Worcestershire sauce
1 slice wholemeal bread
salt and freshly ground
    black pepper

Ingredients for 2

2 tsp olive oil
175g/6oz button mushrooms,
    quartered
2 tsp brown fruity sauce
2 tsp tomato ketchup
1 tsp Worcestershire sauce
2 slices wholemeal bread
salt and freshly ground
    black pepper

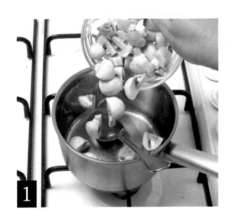

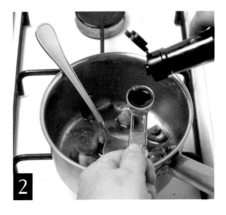

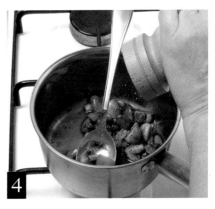

1 Heat the oil in a small pan and sauté the mushrooms for 2–3 minutes until softened and beginning to turn golden.

2 Stir in the fruity sauce, tomato ketchup and Worcestershire sauce and cook gently for a minute or two.

3 Meanwhile lightly toast the bread.

4 Season the mushrooms to taste. Serve on the toast.

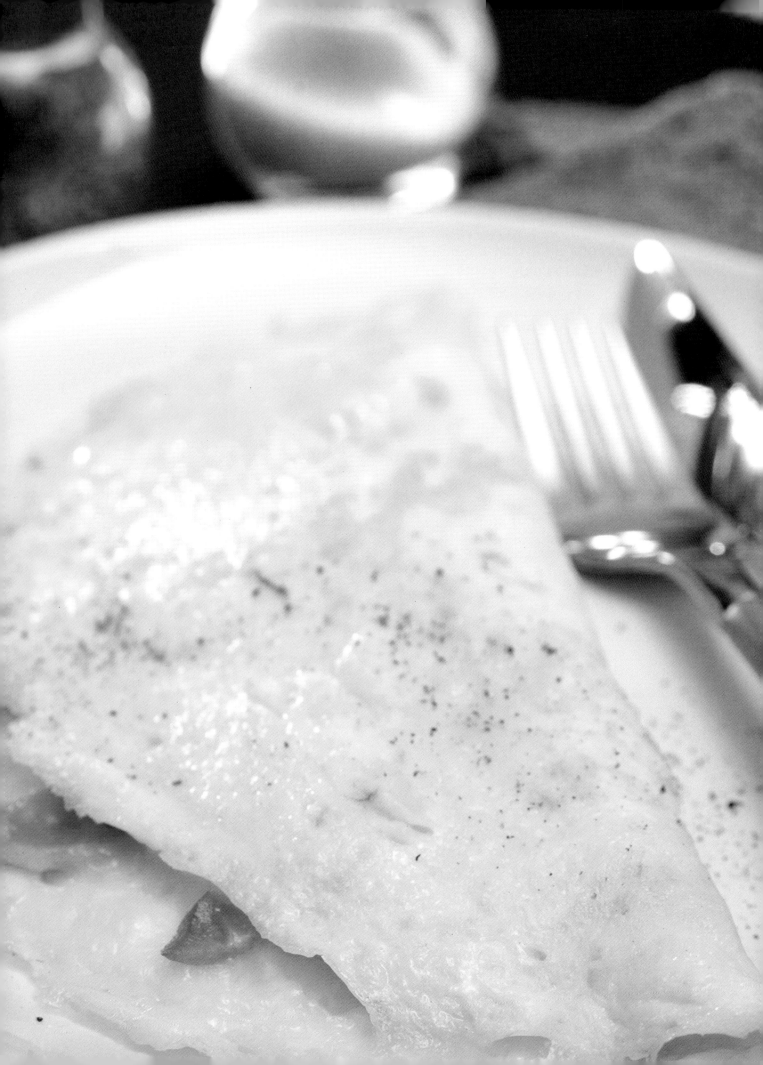

Ham & Cheese Omelette

Omelettes make a great savoury breakfast but it is a good idea not to consume too many eggs in one week as they contain cholesterol which is a contributor to heart disease. Remember, ham can be quite salty so there is no need to add extra salt. Serve with slices of wholemeal toast and grilled tomatoes.

Ingredients for 1

2 eggs
1 tbsp skimmed or semi-skimmed milk
1 tsp olive oil
25g/1oz chopped ham
25g/1oz reduced-fat Cheddar cheese, grated
salt and freshly ground black pepper
pinch of freshly grated nutmeg

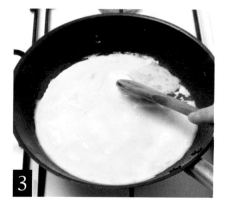

1 Beat the eggs and milk together until slightly frothy. Season with salt, pepper and nutmeg.

2 Heat the oil in a non-stick frying pan, add the egg mixture and cook gently until it begins to set on the bottom.

3 Using a wooden spoon draw in the sides of the omelette and let the egg mixture run to the outside of the pan.

4 Continue until the egg is almost set. Sprinkle the ham and cheese over the surface and allow to cook for a couple more minutes until the cheese begins to melt.

5 Carefully fold the omelette in half and slide out on to a warm serving plate to serve.

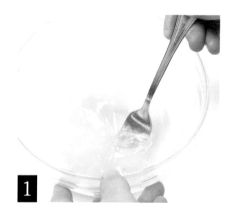

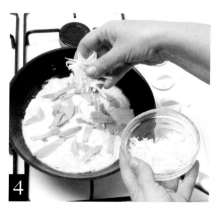

Cheese Toastie

Family Favourite

Easy to make and delicious – a great start to the day. I like to use a tomato relish or chutney but fruity pickle also works well. Serve with grilled tomatoes if liked.

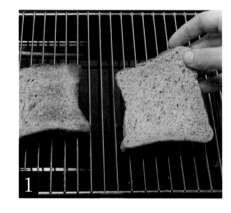

Ingredients for 1

1 slice wholemeal bread
2 tsp tomato relish
40g/1½oz reduced-fat Cheddar cheese or other hard cheese, grated

Ingredients for 2

2 slices wholemeal bread
4 tsp tomato relish
75g/3oz reduced-fat Cheddar cheese or other hard cheese, grated

1 Lightly toast the bread under a medium grill.

2 Spread the relish over the toast.

3 Sprinkle the cheese on top.

4 Place under the grill until the cheese melts. Serve immediately.

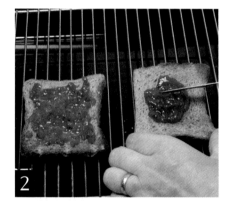

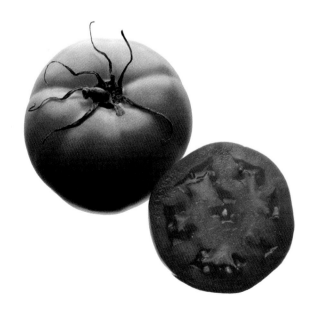

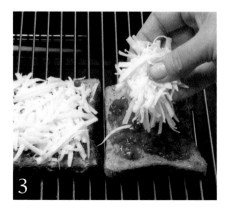

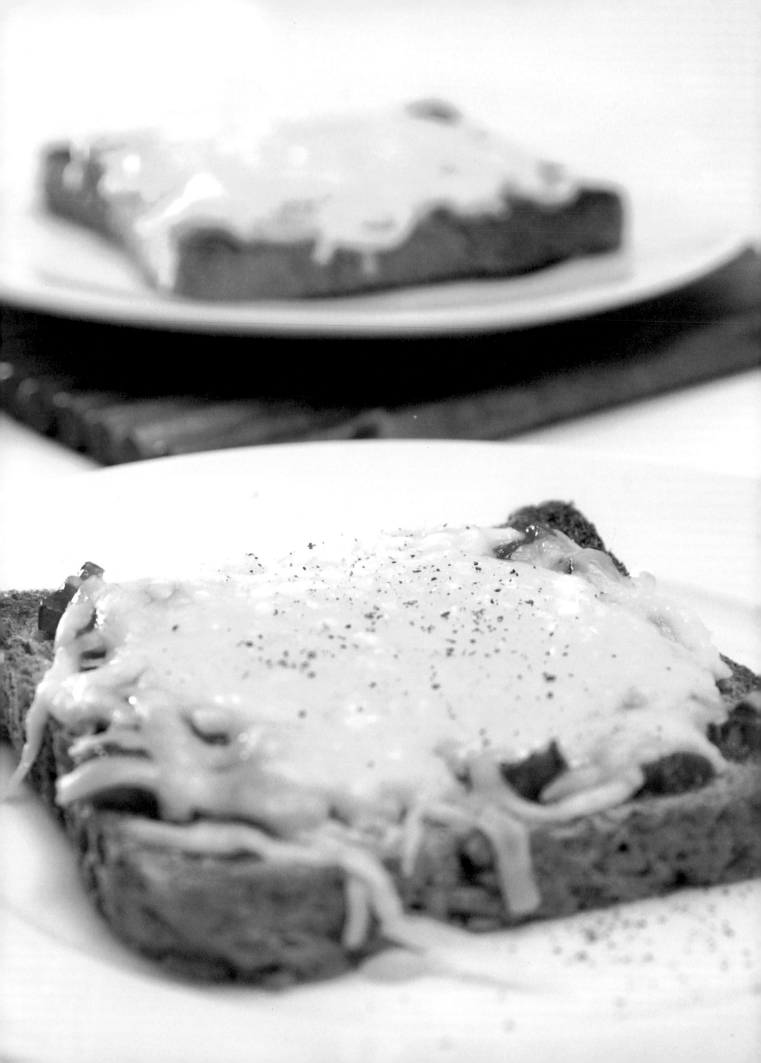

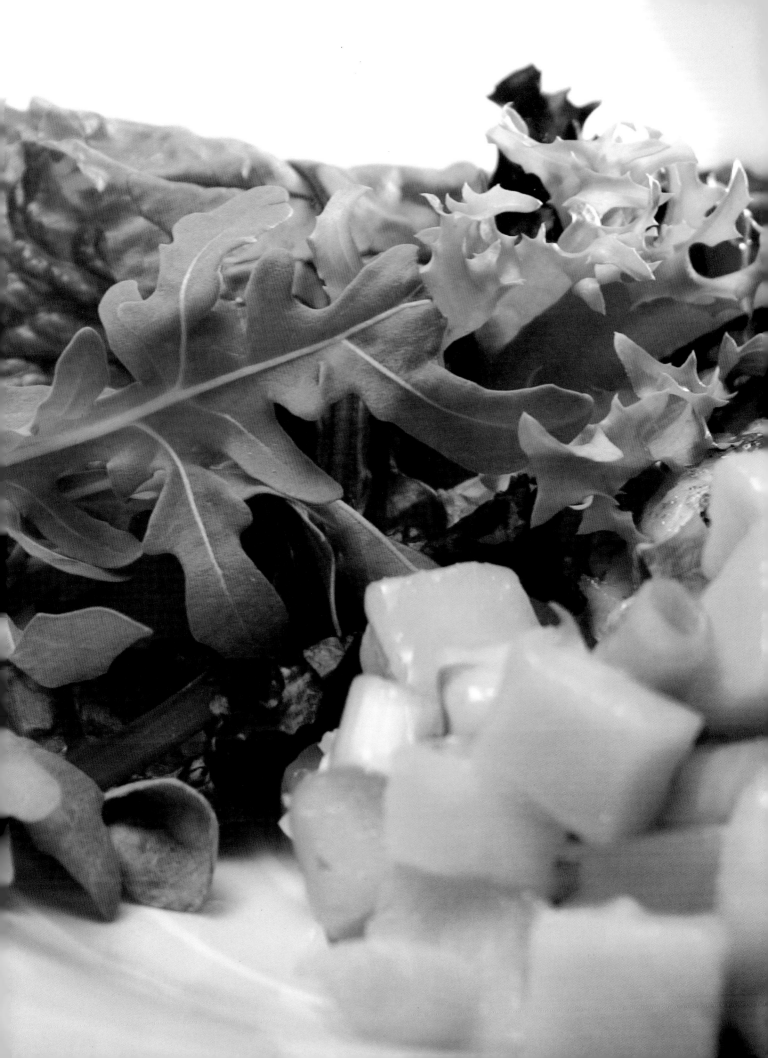

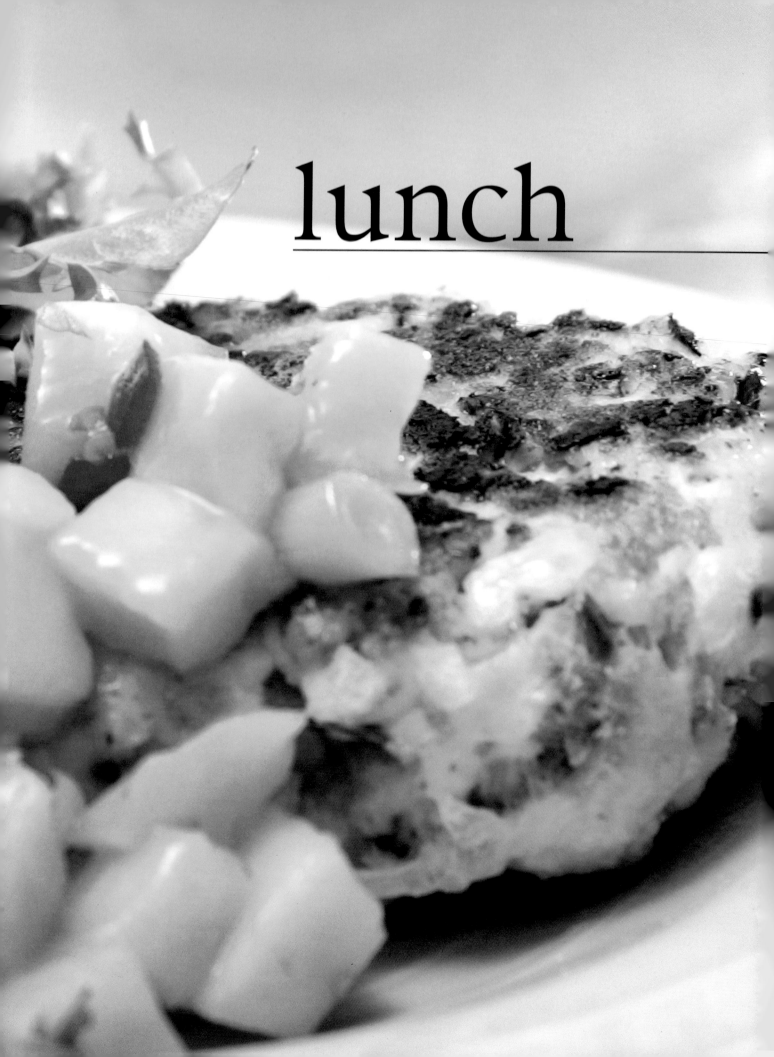

lunch

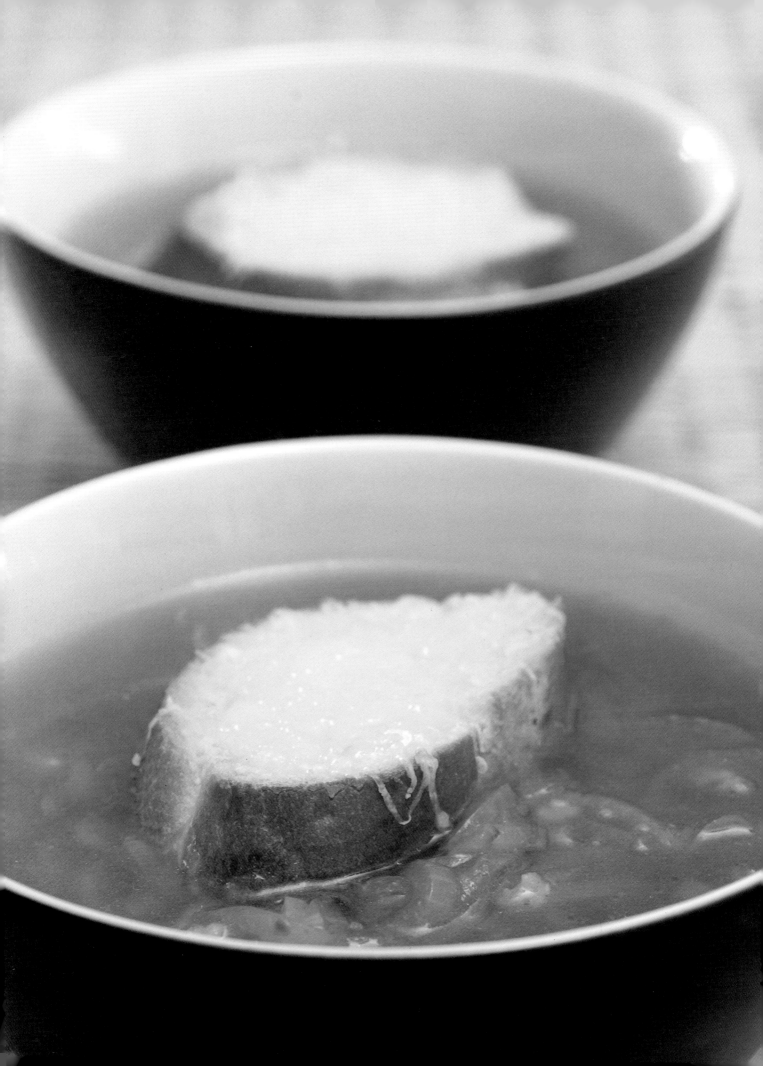

Onion Soup

Easy Entertaining

I have added some brown rice to this traditional soup to increase the carbohydrate content of the dish, but it is still a good idea to serve the soup with extra bread too.

Ingredients for 2

2 tsp olive oil
225g/8oz mild onions, sliced
600ml/1pt good beef or
   vegetable stock
25g/1oz brown rice
1 bay leaf
2 sprigs thyme
2 sprigs parsley
2 slices French bread
15g/½oz Gruyère cheese,
   grated

Ingredients for 4

4 tsp olive oil
450g/1lb mild onions, sliced
1.2l/2pt good beef or
   vegetable stock
50g/2oz brown rice
2 bay leaf
4 sprigs thyme
4 sprigs parsley
4 slices French bread
25g/1oz Gruyère cheese,
   grated

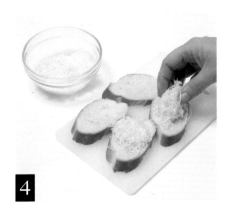

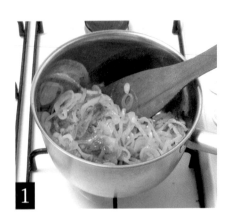

1 Heat the oil in a large saucepan and gently sauté the onions for 10–20 minutes, stirring frequently to prevent them burning. The onions should turn a pale golden colour.

2 Pour in the stock and bring to the boil. Stir in the rice. Tie the herbs together to form a bouquet garni and add to the soup.

3 Reduce the heat, cover and simmer gently for 30 minutes.

4 Remove the bouquet garni. Sprinkle the cheese over the bread slices and place under a preheated grill until the cheese melts and bubbles.

5 Spoon the soup into warm serving bowls and float the cheesy toasts on top.

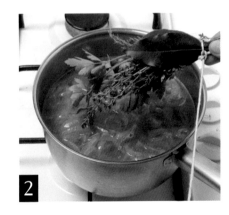

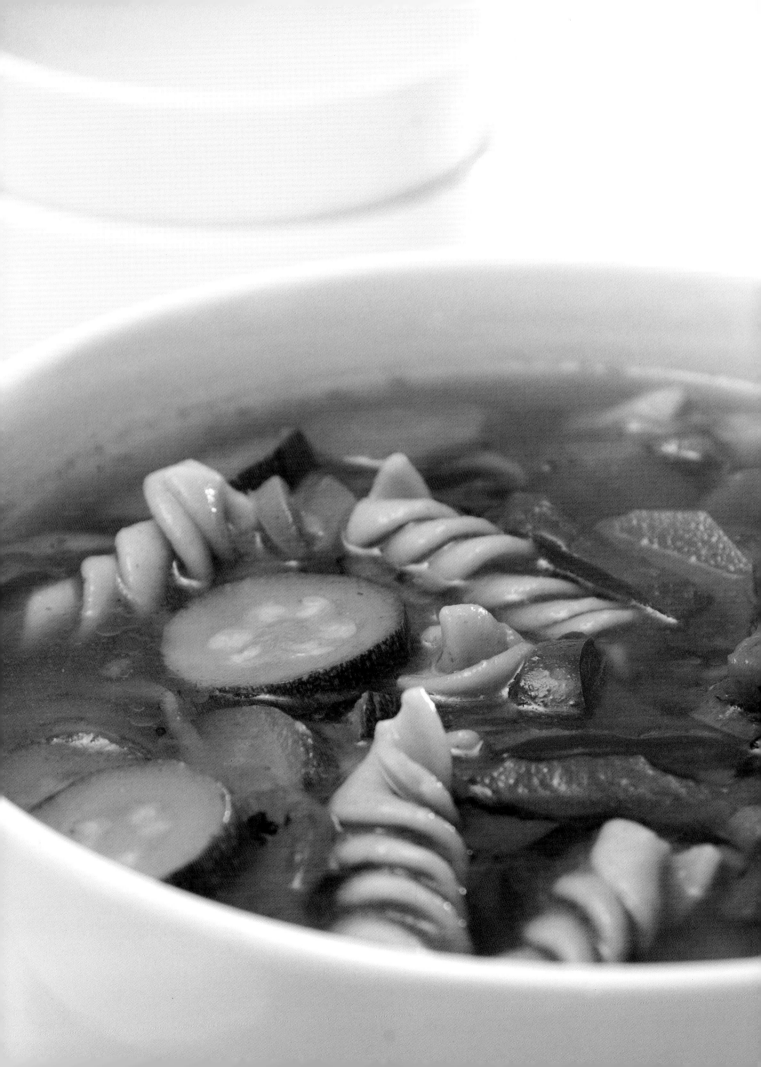

Bean & Pasta Soup

Freezer Friendly

Packed full of vegetables, with beans that provide soluble fibre and wholemeal pasta which provides carbohydrate, this soup is a well-balanced meal for people with diabetes. Why not double the quantities and freeze in usable amounts for a handy meal at any time? Defrost, then reheat gently over a low heat, or in the microwave.

Ingredients for 3

1 tbsp olive oil
1 carrot, sliced
½ small onion, sliced
½ red pepper, seeded and
    sliced
1 small courgette, sliced
50g/2oz mushrooms, sliced
900ml/1½pt vegetable stock
200g/7oz can mixed beans,
    rinsed and drained
50g/2oz wholemeal pasta
    spirals
1 tsp mixed herbs
salt and freshly ground
    black pepper

Ingredients for 6

1 tbsp olive oil
2 carrots, sliced
1 onion, sliced
1 red pepper, seeded and
    sliced
2 small courgettes, sliced
100g/4oz mushrooms, sliced
1.7l/3pt vegetable stock
400g/14oz can mixed beans,
    rinsed and drained
100g/4oz wholemeal pasta
    spirals
2 tsp mixed herbs
salt and freshly ground
    black pepper

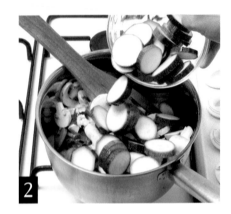
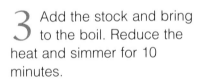
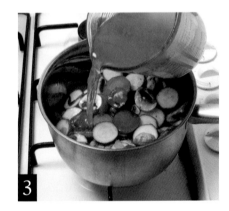

1 Heat the oil in a large saucepan and fry the carrots, onions and peppers over a high heat, stirring for 5 minutes until softened.

2 Add the courgettes and mushrooms and fry for 2 minutes.

3 Add the stock and bring to the boil. Reduce the heat and simmer for 10 minutes.

4 Add the beans and pasta, Bring back to the boil, then stir in the herbs and season to taste. Simmer for 15 minutes. Serve with crusty bread.

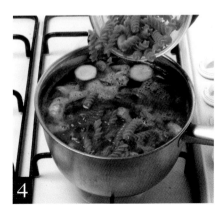

Butterbean & Cumin Soup

vegetarian

This is filling and warming – ideal for a winter lunch. Serve with crusty wholemeal bread. If the soup is too thick you can add a little extra stock. If serving to non-vegetarians you could add some diced ham to the puréed soup.

Ingredients for 2

100g/4oz dried butter beans
1 tsp olive oil
1 small onion, chopped
1 large carrot, chopped
600ml/1pt vegetable stock
½ tsp ground cumin
a little low-fat natural
 yoghurt (optional)
salt and freshly ground
 black pepper

Ingredients for 4

225g/8oz dried butter beans
2 tsp olive oil
1 onion, chopped
2 large carrots, chopped
1.2l/2pt vegetable stock
1 tsp ground cumin
a little low-fat natural
 yoghurt (optional)
salt and freshly ground
 black pepper

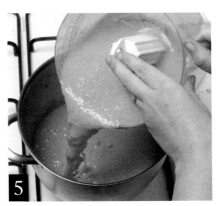

1

1 Rinse the beans and place in a large bowl. Cover with water and leave to soak for at least 12 hours or overnight. Drain.

2 Heat the oil in a large saucepan and fry the onion and carrot for 5 minutes until beginning to soften.

3 Add the beans, stock and cumin. Bring to the boil. Reduce the heat and simmer for 1 hour until the beans are tender.

4 Purée the soup in a liquidiser and season to taste.

5 Return to the pan and reheat gently, stirring. Serve in warm soup bowls with a swirl of yoghurt if desired.

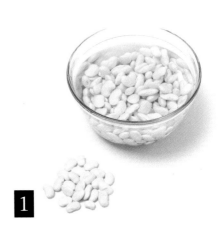

3

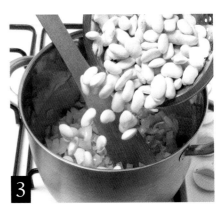

5

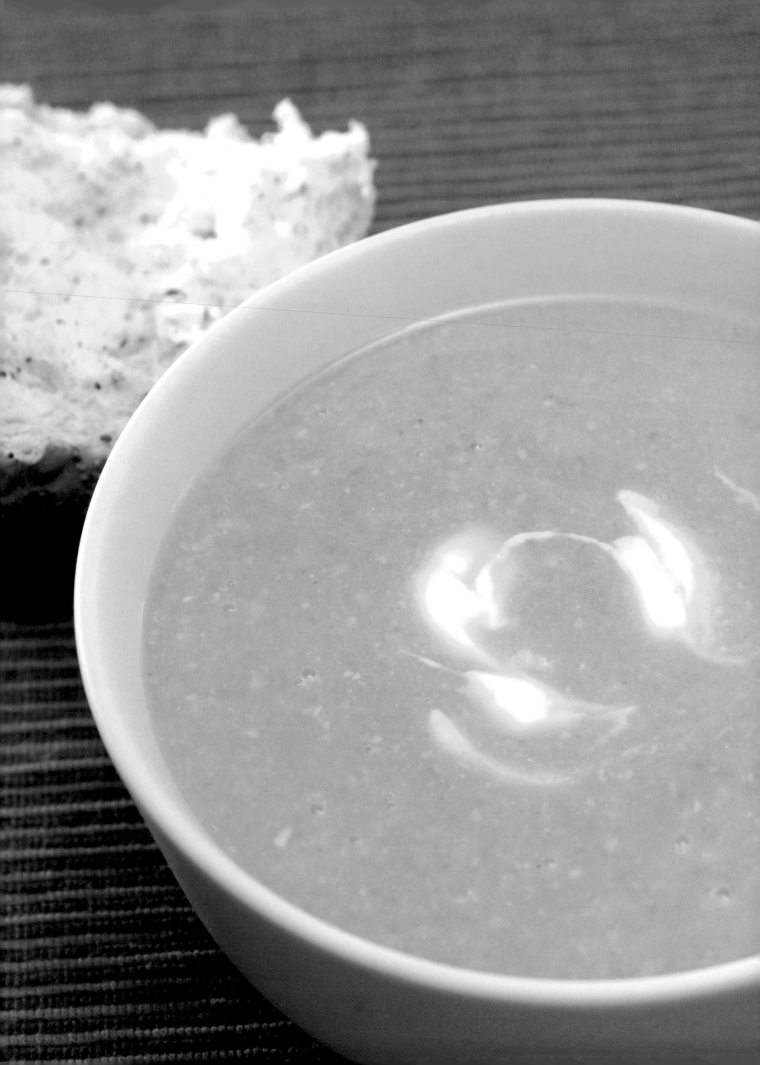

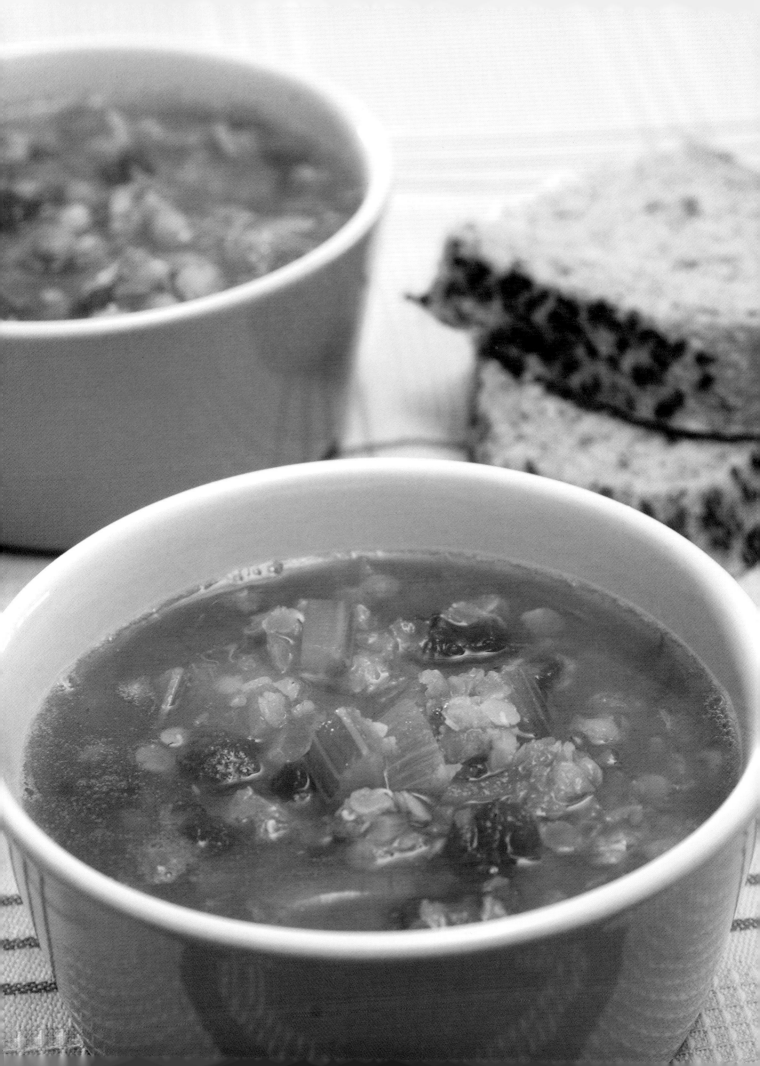

Red Lentil Soup

vegetarian

Pulses such as lentils are great for people with diabetes as they are a good source of soluble fibre which helps even out blood glucose levels. I like to serve this soup with naan bread, but you could also serve it with crusty brown bread.

Ingredients for 2

1 tbsp olive oil
1 small onion, chopped
1 clove garlic, chopped
1 stick celery, chopped
½ tsp each cumin, coriander
  and chilli
75g/3oz red lentils
450ml/¾pt vegetable stock
200g/7oz can chopped
  tomatoes
salt and freshly ground
  black pepper

Ingredients for 4

2 tbsp olive oil
1 onion, chopped
1 clove garlic, chopped
2 sticks celery, chopped
1 tsp each cumin, coriander
  and chilli
175g/6oz red lentils
900ml/1½pt vegetable stock
400g/14oz can chopped
  tomatoes
salt and freshly ground
  black pepper

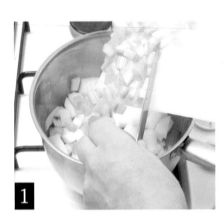

1 Heat the oil in a large saucepan and fry the onion, garlic and celery for 5–10 minutes until softened and just beginning to colour.

2 Add the spices.

3 Rinse the lentils and add to the pan with the stock and tomatoes. Bring to the boil, then reduce the heat and cook covered for 40 minutes.

4 Serve the soup chunky. Alternatively, purée it, return to the pan to reheat and season to taste.

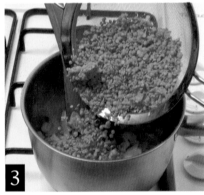

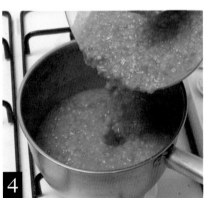

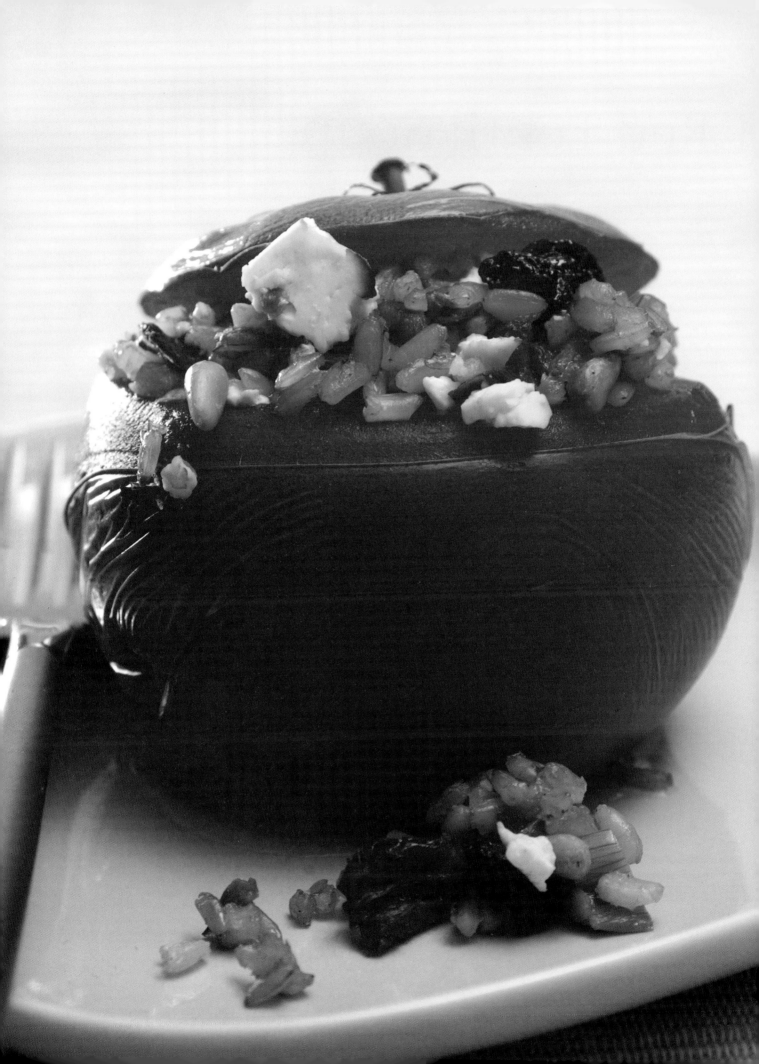

Stuffed Tomatoes with Rice & Pine Nuts

vegetarian

In the summer I prepare this dish up to step 5 using the smaller tomatoes and serve the tomatoes uncooked, accompanied with a green salad and crusty bread. On colder days I prefer to use beefsteak tomatoes and serve this dish hot, accompanied with green beans or broccoli.

Ingredients for 2

2 beefsteak tomatoes or 4
   medium tomatoes
1 tsp olive oil
4 spring onions, sliced
1 clove garlic, crushed
60g/2½oz long grain
   brown rice
150ml/¼pt vegetable stock
1 tbsp chopped fresh
   oregano or 1 tsp dried
   oregano
1 piece sun-dried tomato in
   oil, chopped
25g/1oz feta cheese,
   crumbled
1 tbsp pine nuts, toasted
15g/½oz raisins
salt and freshly ground
   black pepper

Ingredients for 4

4 beefsteak tomatoes or 8
   medium tomatoes
2 tsp olive oil
8 spring onions, sliced
1 clove garlic, crushed
150g/5oz long grain
   brown rice
300ml/½pt vegetable stock
2 tbsp chopped fresh
   oregano or 2 tsp dried
   oregano
2 pieces sun-dried tomatoes
   in oil, chopped
50g/2oz feta cheese,
   crumbled
2 tbsp pine nuts, toasted
25g/1oz raisins
salt and freshly ground
   black pepper

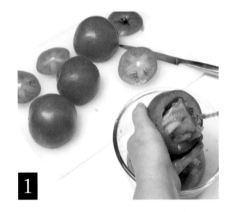

1

1 Slice the tops off the tomatoes and scoop out the flesh and seeds into a bowl. Remove the tomato flesh and chop.

2 Place the tomato shells upside down to drain.

3 Heat the oil in a saucepan and fry the onions and garlic for 2 minutes. Stir in the rice and fry for 1 minute.

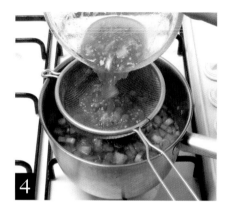

4 Add the stock, tomato flesh, oregano and sun-dried tomatoes. Bring to the boil. Strain in the tomato juice from the seeds. Reduce the heat and simmer covered for 25 minutes until the stock has been absorbed and the rice is tender.

5 Stir in the remaining ingredients. If serving cold allow to cool. Pile the rice mixture into the tomato shells and place lids on top.

6 To serve hot, bake the stuffed tomatoes in a preheated oven 180°C/ 350°F/gas mark 4 for 10–15 minutes.

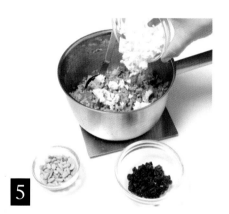

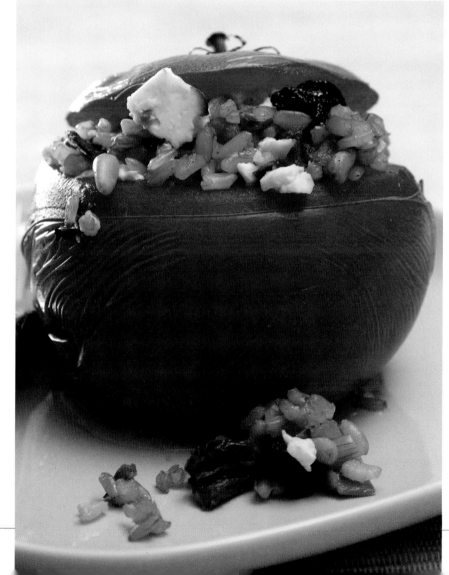

Summer Vegetable Quiche

Prepare Ahead

Quiches are perfect for picnics, packed lunches or summer lunches at home. Serve with a little green salad. Brush baked pastry cases with a little beaten egg while still hot to seal the pastry and prevent leaks. The pastry in this recipe uses a slightly smaller fat to flour ratio than a standard short-crust pastry.

Ingredients for 6

150g/5oz plain flour
100g/4oz plain wholemeal flour
75g/3oz butter or sunflower margarine
a little cold water
75g/3oz asparagus tips, trimmed
75g/3oz baby carrots
50g/2oz frozen petit pois
1 small courgette, sliced
100g/4oz firm goat's cheese, sliced
3 eggs
100g/4oz low-fat crème fraîche
100ml/3¼fl oz skimmed or semi-skimmed milk
salt and freshly ground black pepper
1 tbsp fresh parsley, chopped

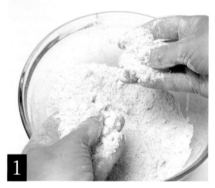

1

1 Place the flour into a bowl, cut the fat into small chunks and rub in with your finger tips until the mixture resembles fine breadcrumbs. Add enough water to mix to a firm dough.

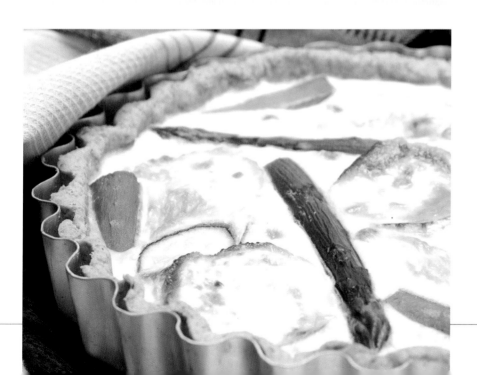

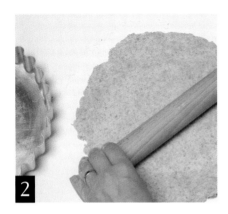

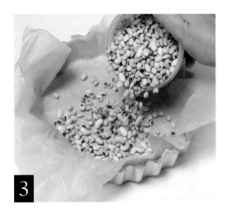

2 Roll out the pastry and use to line a 23cm/9in flan dish or tin. Prick the base all over and chill for 15 minutes.

3 Preheat the oven to 200°C/400°F/gas mark 6. Line the pastry case with baking parchment or greaseproof paper and fill with baking beans.

4 Bake blind for 10 minutes, remove beans and paper and bake for 10 minutes. Reduce the oven temperature to 180°C/350°F/gas mark 4.

5 Meanwhile blanch the asparagus and carrots in boiling water for 3 minutes, add the petit pois and drain.

6 Spread all the vegetables in the pastry case and arrange the cheese on top.

7 Whisk together the eggs, crème fraîche and milk. Season well with salt and pepper. Stir in the parsley. Pour into the pastry case.

8 Bake for 35–40 minutes or until the filling is set and golden.

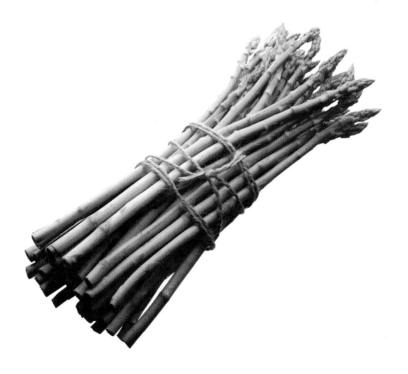

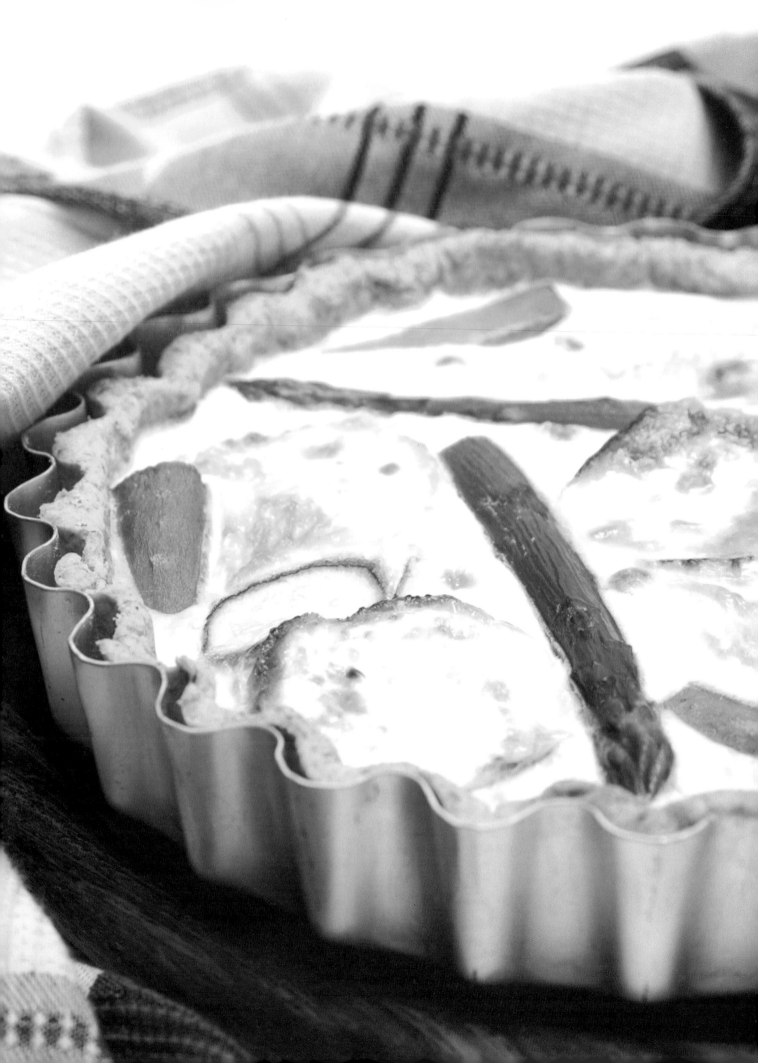

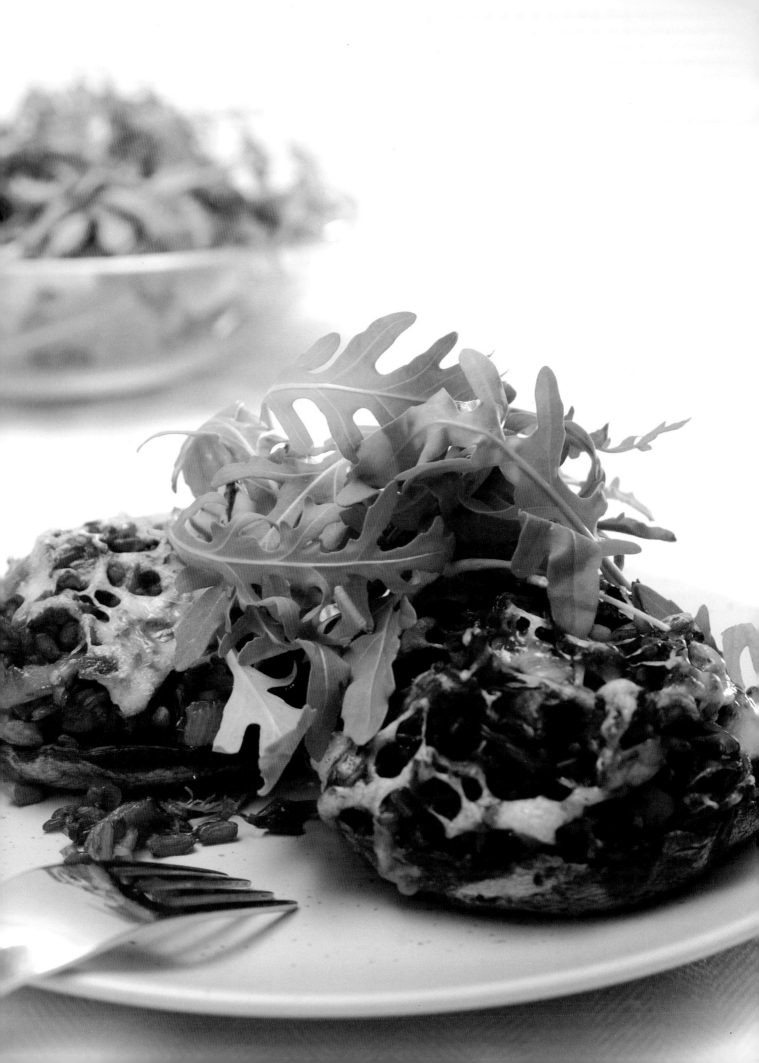

Stuffed Mushrooms

vegetarian

These make a great light meal but you can also halve the quantities and serve as a starter to a main meal. The Camargue red rice has a delicious distinctive nutty flavour. It is available from delis and large supermarkets. Substitute short grain or easy-cook brown rice if you can not find it. Serve with rocket and crusty bread.

Ingredients for 2

225ml/8fl oz vegetable stock
60g/2½oz Camargue red rice
4 large field mushrooms
1 tsp olive oil
½ small red onion
1 clove garlic, chopped
4 tbsp fresh parsley,
   chopped
salt and freshly ground
   black pepper
25g/1oz Edam cheese, grated
rocket leaves to serve

Ingredients for 4

450ml/¾pt vegetable stock
125g/4½oz Camargue red rice
8 large field mushrooms
2 tsp olive oil
1 small red onion
2 cloves garlic, chopped
4 tbsp fresh parsley,
   chopped
salt and freshly ground
   black pepper
50g/2oz Edam cheese, grated
rocket leaves to serve

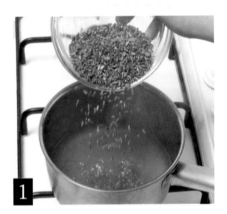

1 Bring the stock to the boil in a small saucepan. Add the rice and stir, then cover and simmer for about 35 minutes. Remove lid and cook for a further minute or two until all the stock has been absorbed.

2 Preheat the oven to 200°C/400°F/gas mark 6. Remove the stalks from the mushrooms and chop finely.

3 Place the mushrooms on a lightly greased baking sheet.

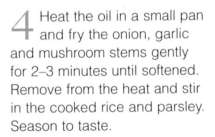

4 Heat the oil in a small pan and fry the onion, garlic and mushroom stems gently for 2–3 minutes until softened. Remove from the heat and stir in the cooked rice and parsley. Season to taste.

5 Spoon the rice mixture on to the mushrooms and sprinkle the cheese on top.

6 Bake for 20–25 minutes until tender. Serve with rocket leaves piled on top.

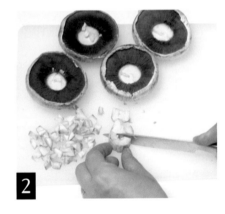

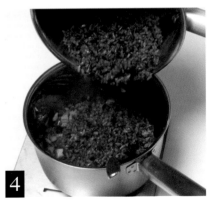

Curried Pasta Salad

Prepare Ahead

This pasta salad is tossed in a yoghurt dressing that is lower in fat than mayonnaise. It is a main meal salad which is ideal for packed lunches.

Ingredients for 2

100g/4oz wholemeal pasta
150g/5oz cooked chicken, cut into bite-size pieces
½ green pepper, seeded and sliced
½ red pepper, seeded and sliced
2 sticks celery, sliced
3 spring onions, sliced
3 tbsp sweetcorn niblets, thawed if frozen
75g/3oz low-fat Greek-style yoghurt
1 tsp hot or medium curry paste
25g/1oz cashew nuts, roasted
salt

Ingredients for 4

225g/8oz wholemeal pasta
300g/10½oz cooked chicken, cut into bite-sized pieces
1 small green pepper, seeded and sliced
1 red pepper, seeded and sliced
4 sticks celery, sliced
6 spring onions, sliced
6 tbsp sweetcorn niblets, thawed if frozen
150g/5oz low-fat Greek-style yoghurt
2 tsp hot or medium curry paste
50g/2oz cashew nuts, roasted
salt

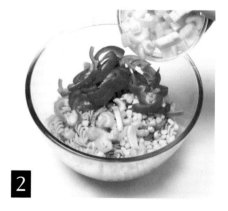

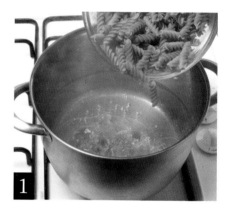

1 Cook the pasta in plenty of lightly salted boiling water for 12 minutes, or as directed on the packet.

2 Drain and place in a large bowl. Add the chicken, peppers, celery, onions and sweetcorn and toss to combine.

3 Mix together the yoghurt and curry paste.

4 Drizzle the dressing over the salad. Scatter the nuts on top. Just before serving, toss to coat in the dressing.

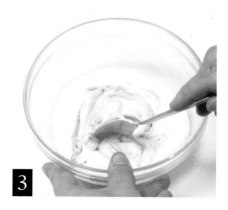

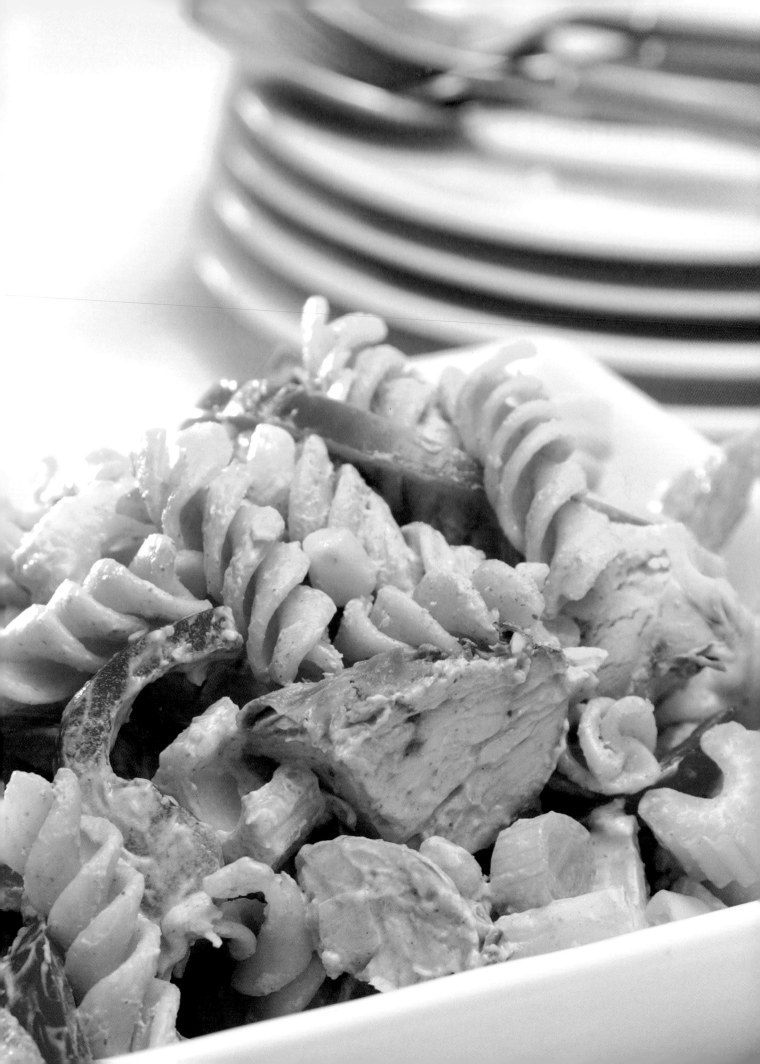

Spanish Tortilla

This is a versatile lunch dish which is fantastic served either hot or cold. You can vary the vegetables you add. If I do not have fresh peppers to hand I often use diced frozen vegetables (thawed) instead. Serve with a green salad and fresh bread.

Ingredients for 2

2 tsp olive oil
½ small onion, chopped
100g/4oz left-over cooked potatoes, cut into small dice
¼ red pepper, seeded and chopped
¼ green pepper, seeded and chopped
50g/2oz ham, sliced into small strips
3 eggs
1 tbsp skimmed or semi-skimmed milk
salt and freshly ground black pepper
pinch of grated nutmeg

Ingredients for 4

1 tbsp olive oil
1 small onion, chopped
225g/8oz left-over cooked potatoes, cut into small dice
½ red pepper, seeded and chopped
½ green pepper, seeded and chopped
100g/4oz ham, sliced into small strips
6 eggs
2 tbsp skimmed milk or semi-skimmed milk
salt and freshly ground black pepper
pinch of grated nutmeg

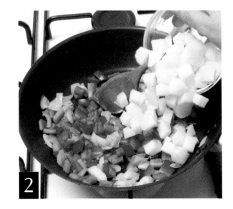

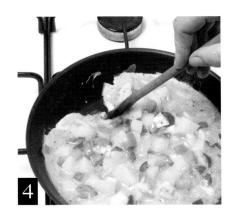

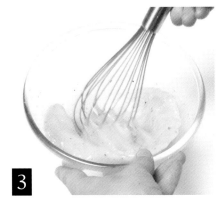

1 Heat the olive oil in an 18cm/7in (20cm/8in) non-stick frying pan. Add the onion and sauté over a medium heat for about 5–10 minutes until softened.

2 Add the potato and peppers and cook for a further 10 minutes. Stir in the ham. Preheat the grill.

3 Beat the eggs, milk, seasoning and nutmeg together with a small hand whisk or fork.

4 Pour the egg mixture into the pan and cook over a low heat. As the mixture begins to set, pull the outside of the egg mixture to the middle and let more run to the outside. Do this once or twice, then leave the pan over a low heat for 2–3 minutes until the underside begins to brown.

5 Place the pan under the preheated grill and allow to cook for a few minutes more until the top is set and golden. Cut into wedges and serve from the pan, or transfer to a plate and allow to cool.

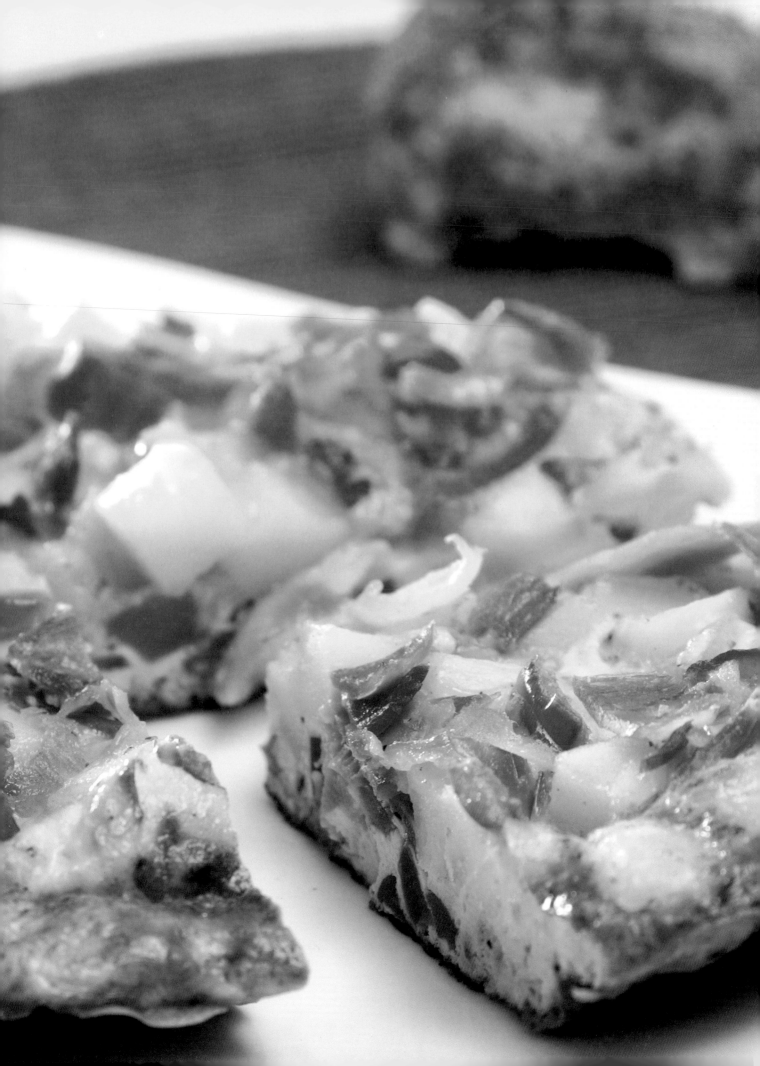

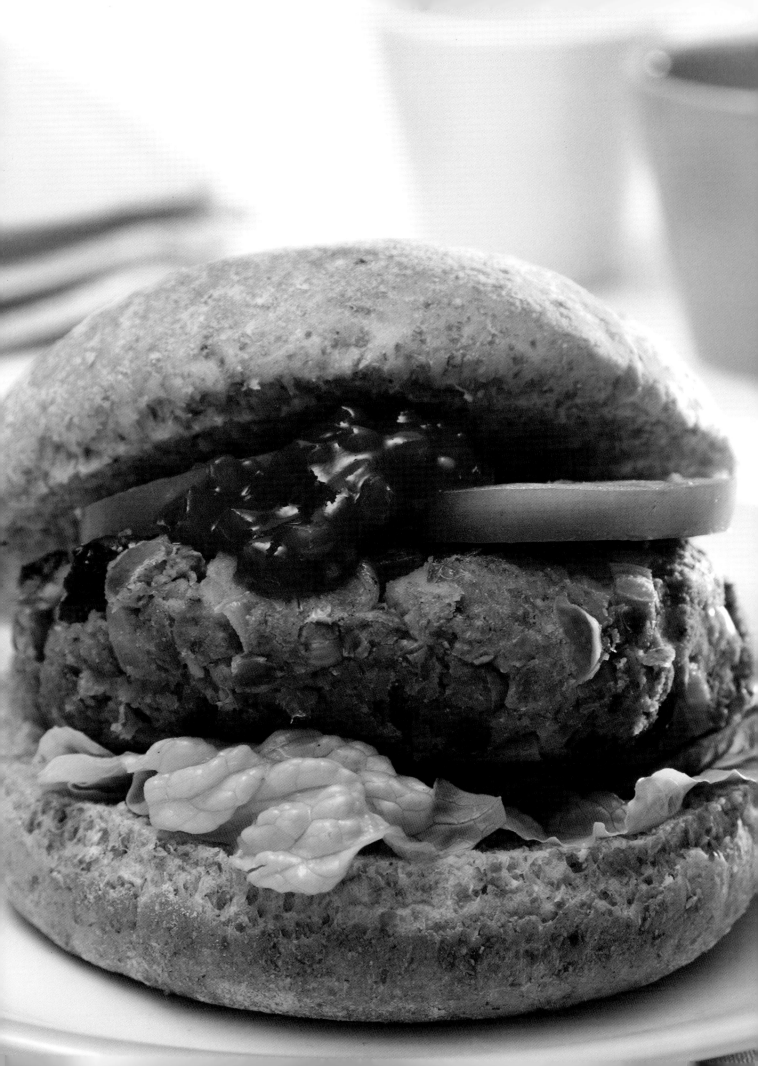

Spicy Bean Burgers

vegetarian

Serve these burgers in wholemeal bread, baps or pitta bread with a little salad.

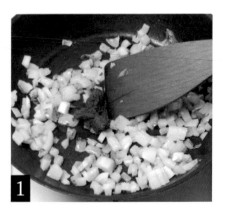

Ingredients for 2

1 tsp sunflower oil, plus a
   little oil for cooking
½ small onion, finely
   chopped
1 stick celery, finely chopped
½ small carrot, finely
   chopped
1 clove garlic, crushed
1 tsp medium or hot curry
   paste
400g/14oz can mixed beans,
   rinsed and drained
50g/2oz wholemeal
   breadcrumbs
a little beaten egg
salt and freshly ground
   black pepper

Ingredients for 4

2 tsp sunflower oil, plus a
   little oil for cooking
1 small onion, finely chopped
2 sticks celery finely
   chopped
1 small carrot, finely
   chopped
2 cloves garlic, crushed
1 tbsp medium or hot curry
   paste
2 x 400g/14oz cans mixed
   beans, rinsed and drained
100g/4oz wholemeal
   breadcrumbs
1 egg
salt and freshly ground
   black pepper

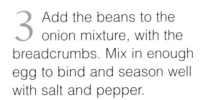

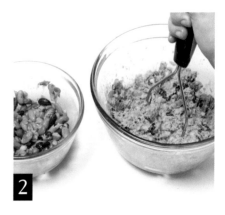

1 Heat the oil and fry the onion, celery, carrot and garlic gently for 5 minutes until softened. Stir in the curry paste.

2 Remove from the heat. Allow to cool. Mash half to three quarters of the beans to a fairly smooth purée and coarsely mash the remaining beans. Mix the beans together.

3 Add the beans to the onion mixture, with the breadcrumbs. Mix in enough egg to bind and season well with salt and pepper.

4 Shape into 2 (4) rounds. Lightly oil a non-stick frying pan. Heat the pan and cook the burgers for 5 minutes each side until crisp and golden.

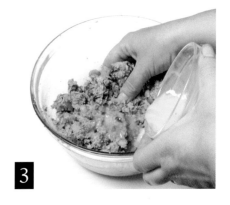

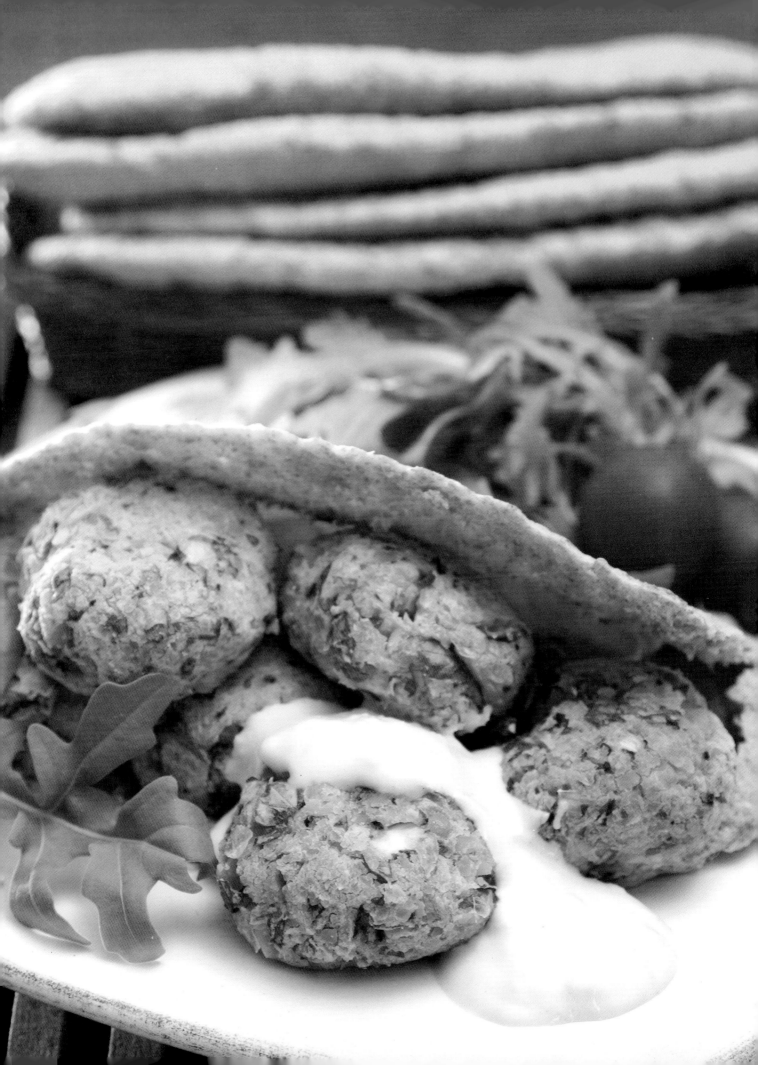

Falafel

vegetarian

These tasty balls are made from chick peas which are a good sauce of calcium and soluble fibre. They are usually fried but here they are baked in the oven to keep the fat content down. They can be eaten hot or cold. Serve with salad and wholemeal pitta bread. They can also be served with natural yoghurt in place of the tahini sauce if preferred.

Makes 12

400g/14oz can chick peas, drained
2 spring onions, chopped
1 clove garlic, chopped
2 tbsp water
2 tbsp flat leaf parsley, chopped
2 tbsp fresh coriander, chopped
½ tsp ground cumin
salt and freshly ground black pepper
1 tbsp sunflower oil

Tahini sauce:

2 tbsp tahini
1 small clove garlic, crushed
1 tbsp lemon juice
1-2 tbsp water

Makes 24

2 x 400g/14oz cans chick peas, drained
4 spring onions, chopped
2 cloves garlic, chopped
4 tbsp water
4 tbsp flat leaf parsley, chopped
4 tbsp fresh coriander, chopped
1 tsp ground cumin
salt and freshly ground black pepper
2 tbsp sunflower oil

Tahini sauce:

4 tbsp tahini
1 clove garlic, crushed
2 tbsp lemon juice
2-4 tbsp water

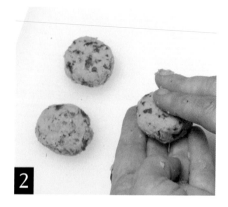

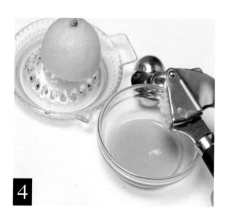

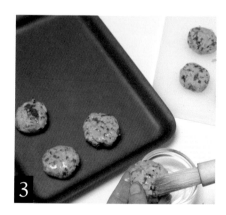

1 Preheat the oven to 190°C/375°F/gas mark 5. Place the chick peas, onion, garlic, water, herbs and cumin in a food processor. Season with salt and pepper.

2 Process to form a smooth purée. Form the mixture into balls about the size of a walnut. Flatten slightly.

3 Brush lightly on all sides with oil and place on a baking sheet. Bake for 15–20 minutes until piping hot.

4 To make the tahini sauce, mix together the tahini, garlic, lemon juice and water to form a runny sauce and season with salt and pepper.

5 Serve the falafel with the tahini sauce drizzled over.

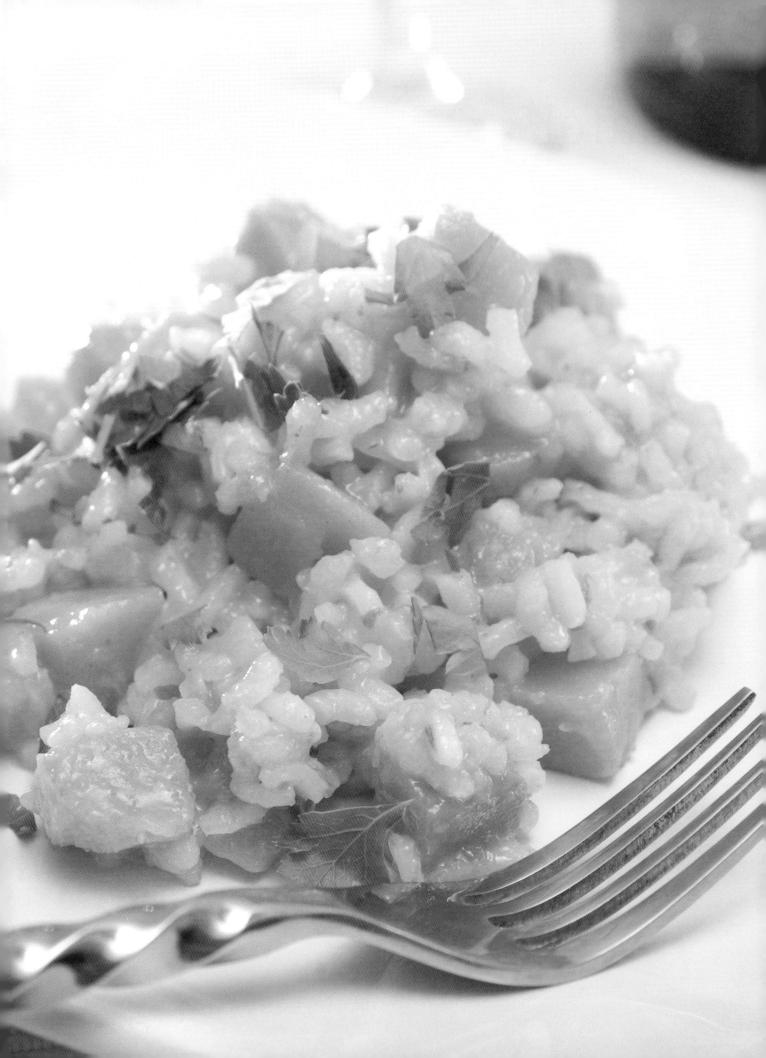

Pumpkin Risotto

One Pot

A traditional risotto has massive amounts of butter and lots of cheese which, while delicious, is packed full of fat and calories. My risotto recipe omits the butter altogether and uses only a little cheese, but the creamy texture of the pumpkin more than makes up for it. Use a good flavoured stock when making risotto, preferably home-made. One medium butternut squash will give about 500g/1lb 2oz of flesh.

Ingredients for 2

- **4 tsp olive oil**
- **150g/5oz pumpkin flesh or butternut squash, cut into small cubes**
- **1 small onion, chopped**
- **1 clove garlic, chopped**
- **125g/4½oz risotto rice**
- **75ml/2½fl oz dry white wine**
- **375ml/13fl oz vegetable or chicken stock**
- **salt and freshly ground black pepper**
- **25g/1oz Parmesan cheese, grated**
- **1 tbsp fresh parsley, chopped**

Ingredients for 4

- **3 tbsp olive oil**
- **500g/1lb 2oz pumpkin or butternut squash, cut into small cubes**
- **1 onion, chopped**
- **2 cloves garlic, chopped**
- **225g/8oz risotto rice**
- **150ml/¼pt dry white wine**
- **750ml/1¼pt vegetable or chicken stock**
- **salt and freshly ground black pepper**
- **50g/2oz Parmesan cheese, grated**
- **2 tbsp fresh parsley, chopped**

1 Heat the oil in a large saucepan and gently sauté the pumpkin or squash for 5–10 minutes, until beginning to soften.

2 Add the onion and garlic and sauté for 5 minutes.

3 Stir in the rice.

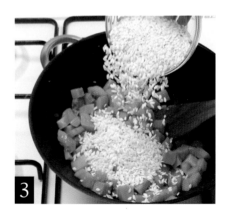

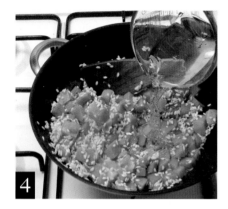

4 Then add the wine.

5 Simmer, stirring occasionally until the wine has been absorbed.

6 Meanwhile heat the stock in a small pan and keep warm. Ladle hot stock into the pan and cook stirring until absorbed.

7 Continue to add the stock a ladleful at a time until all the stock has been absorbed and the rice is tender.

8 Season to taste with salt and pepper. Stir in the Parmesan cheese.

9 Stir in the parsley or sprinkle over the top and serve immediately.

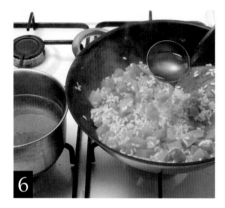

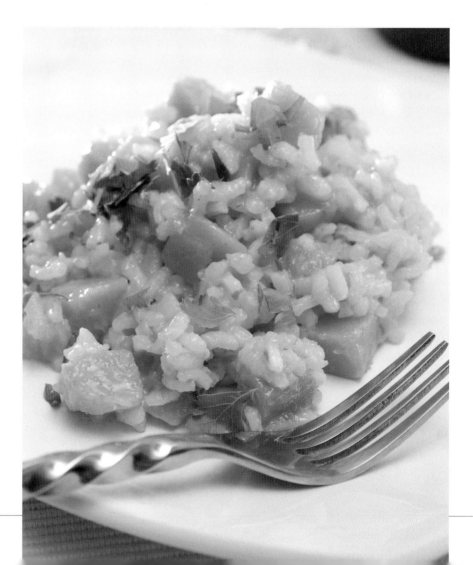

Spinach & Ricotta Filo Pie

vegetarian

Ricotta cheese is a good choice because it is a low-fat cheese. Filo pastry is also much lower in fat than other pastries. Serve this dish hot or cold. It is perfect for packed lunches, served with some cherry tomatoes and some crusty wholemeal bread.

Ingredients for 2

250g/9oz spinach, washed
about 2 tbsp olive oil
1 small onion, chopped
1 clove garlic
125g/4½oz ricotta cheese
1 egg
¼ tsp grated nutmeg
salt and freshly ground
   black pepper
6 sheets filo pastry

Ingredients for 4

500g/1lb 2oz spinach, washed
about 3 tbsp olive oil
1 onion, chopped
2 cloves garlic
250g/9oz ricotta cheese
2 eggs
½ tsp grated nutmeg
salt and freshly ground
   black pepper
6 sheets filo pastry

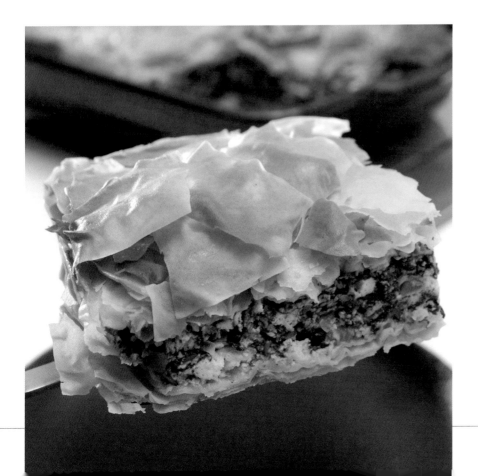

1 Preheat the oven to 190°C/375°F/gas mark 5. Lightly oil a shallow ovenproof dish.

2 Remove any tough stalks from the spinach, and shake excess water from the leaves.

3 Heat 1 tsp (2 tsp) of the oil in a large saucepan and fry the onion gently for 5 minutes until beginning to soften. Add the garlic and fry for 1 minute.

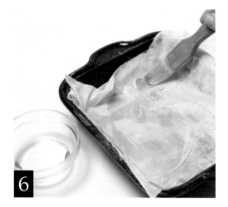

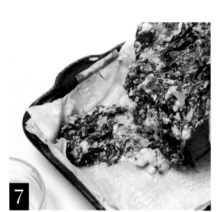

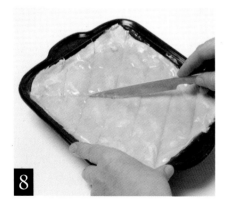

4 Add the spinach to the pan, cover and cook for 4–5 minutes until the spinach has just wilted. Remove from the heat. Drain off any water.

5 Beat the cheese, eggs and nutmeg together and season with salt and pepper. Stir in the spinach.

6 Cut the filo sheets in half. Place one sheet of filo in the ovenproof dish and brush with oil. Layer up the pastry until you have used half of the filo sheets, brushing each layer with a little oil.

7 Spoon the cheese and spinach mixture on top. Fold over the edges of the pastry. Cover with the remaining filo, brushing each layer with oil.

8 Trim the edges of the pastry. Lightly score the top one or two layers of pastry with a knife.

9 Bake for 1 hour until the pastry is golden. Serve hot or cold.

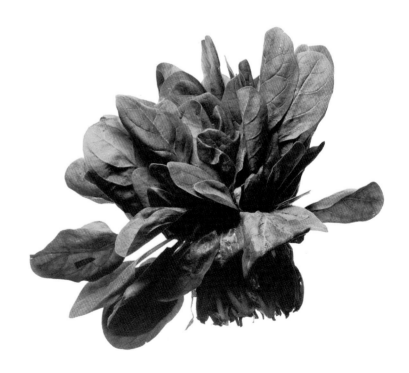

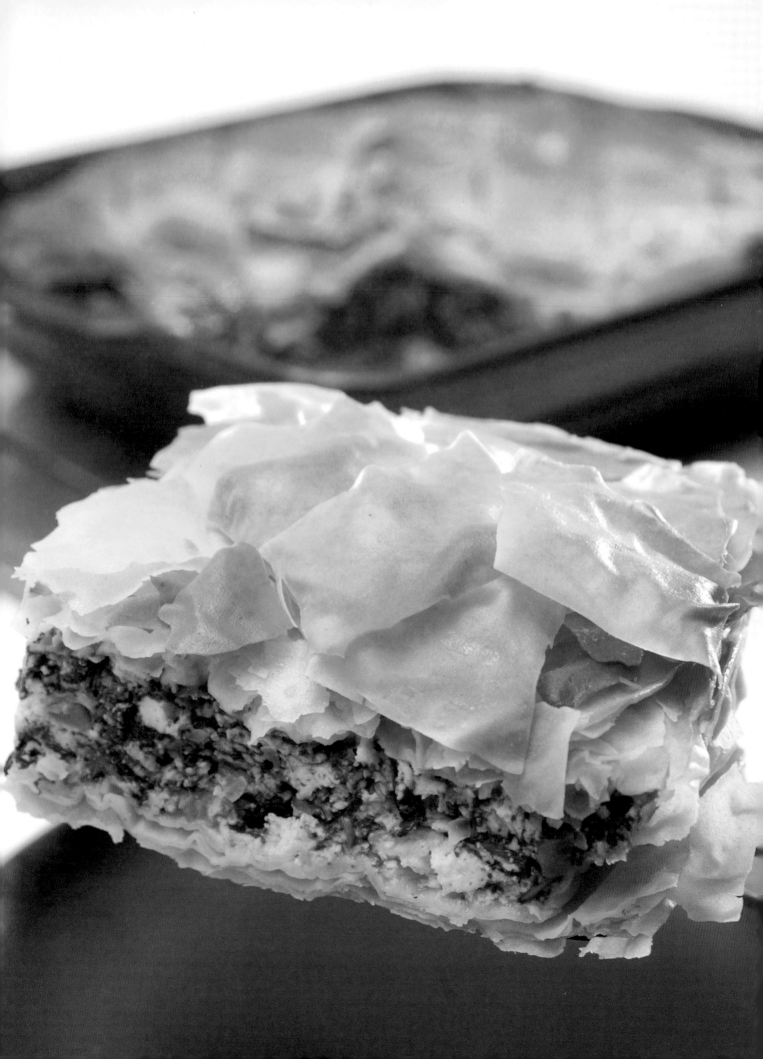

Pumpkin & Nut Loaf

vegetarian

The nuts and seeds give this meat-free loaf a fabulous flavour.

Ingredients for 4

25g/1oz hazelnuts
25g/1oz pistachios
2 tbsp sunflower seeds
1 tsp olive oil
1 small onion, chopped
1 clove garlic
300g/10½oz pumpkin flesh, cubed
75ml/2½fl oz water
25g/1oz fresh wholemeal breadcrumbs
1 egg, lightly beaten
4 tbsp fresh parsley, chopped
salt and freshly ground black pepper
1 tbsp pumpkin seeds

Ingredients for 8

50g/2oz hazelnuts
50g/2oz pistachios
4 tbsp sunflower seeds
2 tsp olive oil
1 large onion, chopped
2 cloves garlic
600g/1lb 5oz pumpkin flesh, cubed
150ml/¼pt water
50g/2oz fresh wholemeal breadcrumbs
2 eggs, lightly beaten
8 tbsp fresh parsley, chopped
salt and freshly ground black pepper
2 tbsp pumpkin seeds

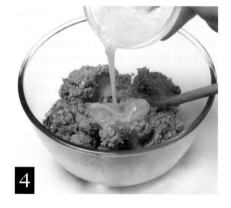

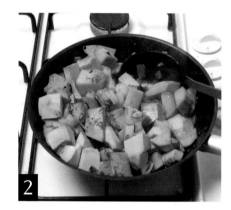

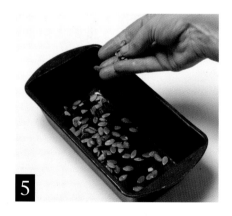

1 Preheat the oven to 190°C/375°F/gas mark 5. Place the hazelnuts, pistachios and sunflower seeds on a baking sheet and roast for 10 minutes until golden.

2 Heat the oil in a small pan and fry the onion and garlic until softened. Stir in the pumpkin and fry for 2–3 minutes. Add the water and simmer for 5 minutes.

3 Place the toasted nuts and seeds in a food processor and coarsely chop. Add the pumpkin and onion mixture and process until combined.

Do not over-process – the mixture should be quite lumpy.

4 Transfer to a bowl and beat in the breadcrumbs, eggs and parsley. Season well.

5 Spread the pumpkin seeds evenly over the base of a lightly greased 450g/1lb (900g/2lb) loaf tin. Spoon the pumpkin and nut mixture into the tin and press down well.

6 Bake for 40–60 minutes. Allow to cool in the tin for 10 minutes before turning out to serve.

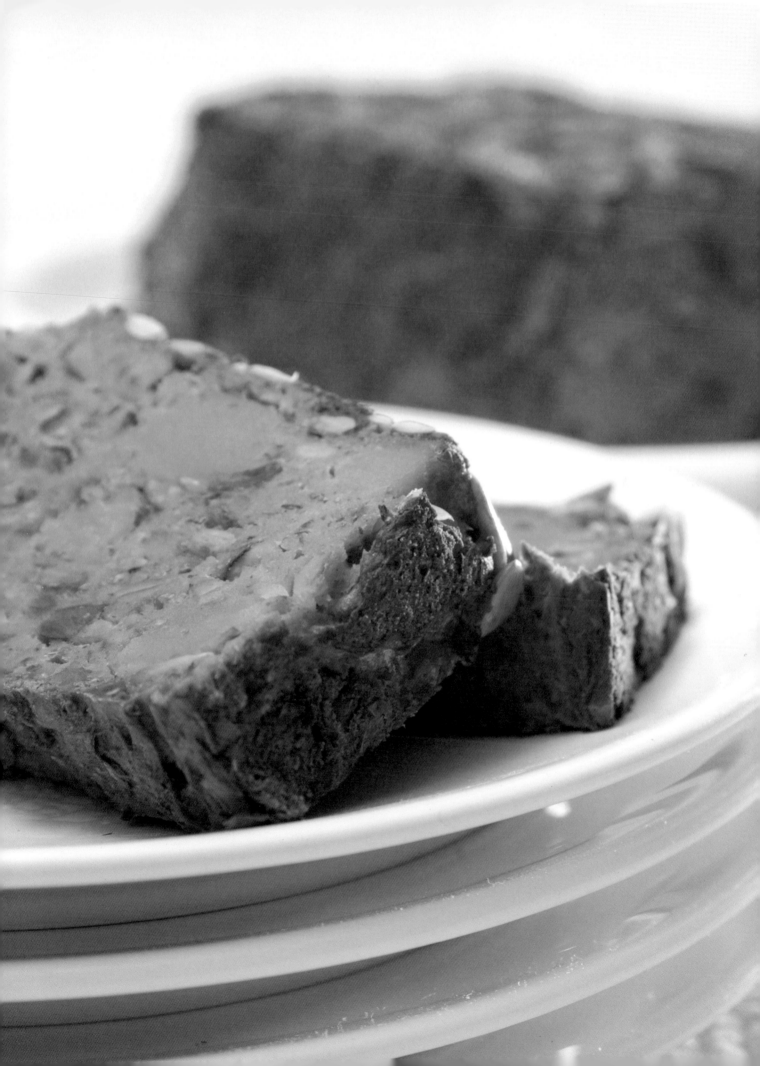

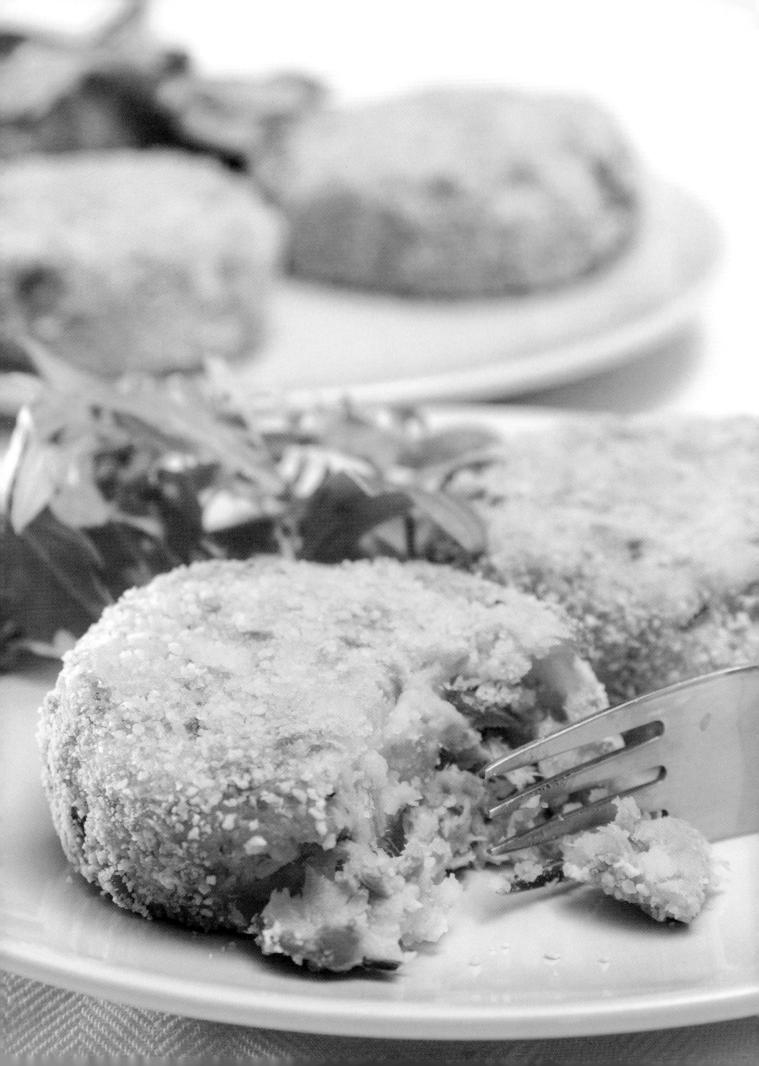

Oven Baked Salmon Fish Cakes

Family Favourite

Fish cakes are usually shallow-fried but they absorb quite a lot of fat when cooked this way. Oven-baked they still have lots of flavour and the fat content is reduced. The bones in canned salmon can be eaten as they are very soft, and they add extra calcium – but remove them if you prefer.

Ingredients for 2

350g/12oz potatoes, peeled
    and cut into small chunks
200g/7oz can pink or red
    salmon, drained
1 tsp chives, snipped
salt and freshly ground
    black pepper
25g/1oz dried breadcrumbs
2 tsp sunflower oil

Ingredients for 4

700g/1½lb potatoes, peeled
    and cut into small chunks
400g/14oz can pink or red
    salmon, drained
1 tbsp chives, snipped
salt and freshly ground
    black pepper
50g/2oz dried breadcrumbs
4 tsp sunflower oil

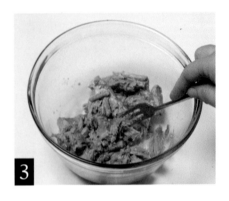

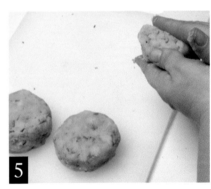

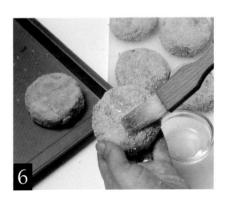

1 Cook the potatoes in lightly salted boiling water for 10–15 minutes until just tender.

2 Preheat the oven to 200°C/400°F/gas mark 6.

3 Drain the salmon and empty into a mixing bowl. Discard the skin and break up the flesh with a fork. Stir in the chives. Season well.

4 Drain the potatoes well, and mash with the fish until well combined.

5 Shape the mixture into 4 (8) rounds. Coat in the breadcrumbs.

6 Lightly brush the cakes with the oil and place on a baking sheet. Bake for 20 minutes until crisp and golden.

7 Serve with salad or green vegetables.

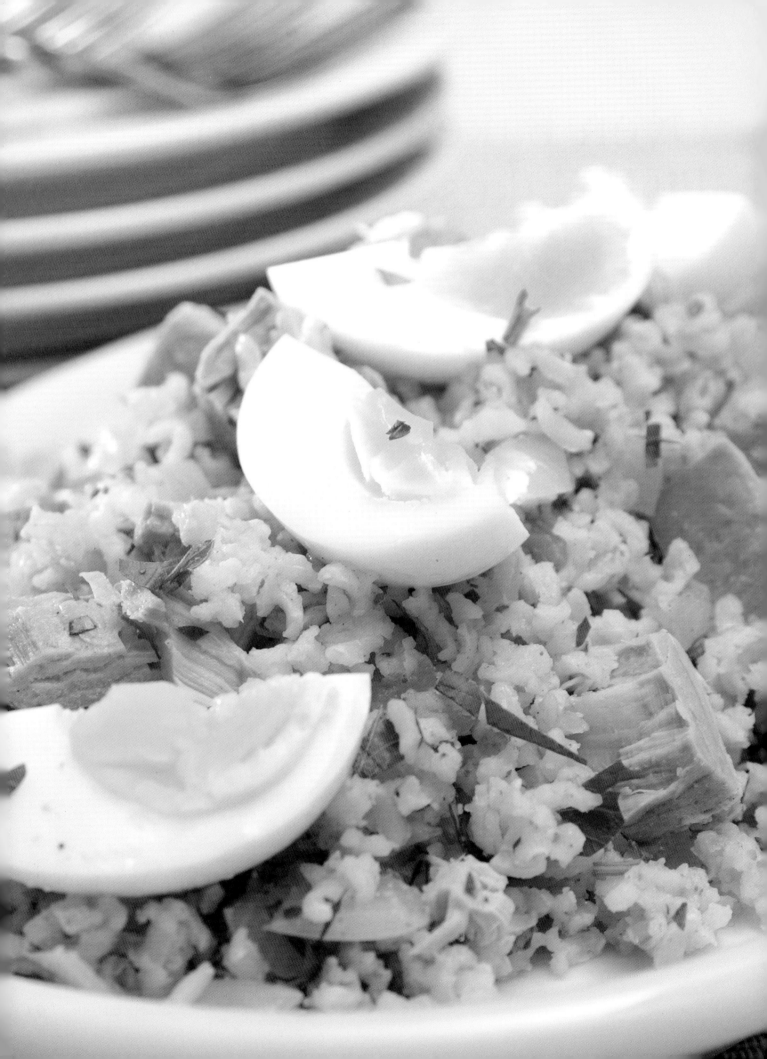

Tuna Kedgeree

I have adapted the traditional kedgeree recipe to create a healthier version. Smoked fish has been replaced with tuna which is an oily fish important for its omega 3 fatty acids, and brown rice adds extra soluble fibre, making this dish perfect for diabetics.

Ingredients for 2

75g/3oz brown basmati rice
100g/4oz fresh tuna
1 tsp sunflower oil
½ small onion, chopped
2 tsp mild curry paste or
    powder
2 tbsp reduced-fat single
    cream (optional)
1 hard-boiled egg, peeled
    and cut into wedges
1 tbsp fresh parsley,
    chopped

Ingredients for 4

175g/6oz brown basmati rice
225g/8oz fresh tuna
2 tsp sunflower oil
1 small onion, chopped
1 tbsp mild curry paste or
    powder
4 tbsp reduced-fat single
    cream (optional)
2 hard-boiled eggs, peeled
    and cut into wedges
2 tbsp fresh parsley,
    chopped

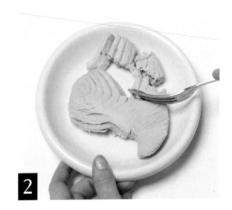

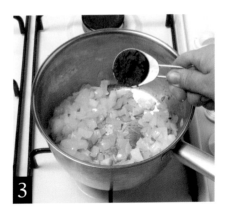

1 Bring a saucepan of water to the boil. Add the rice and stir, then simmer gently for 25 minutes or until the rice is just tender.

2 Meanwhile place the tuna in a non-stick frying pan and cover with cold water. Bring quickly to the boil, then reduce the heat and simmer gently for 5 to 8 minutes. Drain, transfer to a plate and flake the fish into large chunks.

3 In a large saucepan heat the oil and sauté the onion for 3 minutes until softened. Stir in the curry paste and cook gently for another minute.

4 Drain the rice and add to the pan. Stir to coat in the curry mixture. Add the fish and toss gently together, adding the cream if desired.

5 Transfer to a serving dish and top with the hard-boiled egg wedges. Sprinkle with parsley and serve.

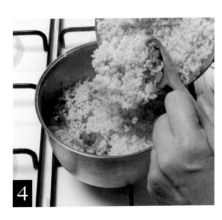

Smoked Fish Paté

Quick and Easy

This is delicious spread on toast, or used to make a sandwich. It can also be served as a dip and with vegetable crudités.

Ingredients for 2

1 kipper
100g/4oz smoked mackerel
100g/4oz reduced-fat Greek-
    style natural yoghurt
1 tbsp fresh chives, snipped
freshly ground black pepper

Ingredients for 4

2 kippers
225g/8oz smoked mackerel
200g/7oz reduced-fat Greek-
    style natural yoghurt
2 tbsp fresh chives, snipped
freshly ground black pepper

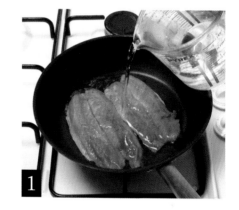

1 Place the kippers in a small non-stick frying pan and add enough water to cover. Bring to the boil, then reduce the heat and simmer gently for 5–8 minutes or until the fish flakes easily. Allow to cool.

2 Flake the kippers and mackerel into a bowl, discarding the skins and any bones. Mash with a fork.

3 Add the yoghurt and chives. Season with pepper.

4 Mix until well combined.

5 Spoon into a serving dish and chill until required.

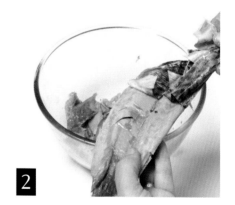

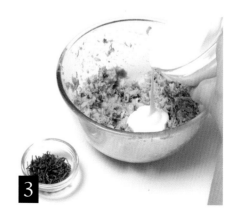

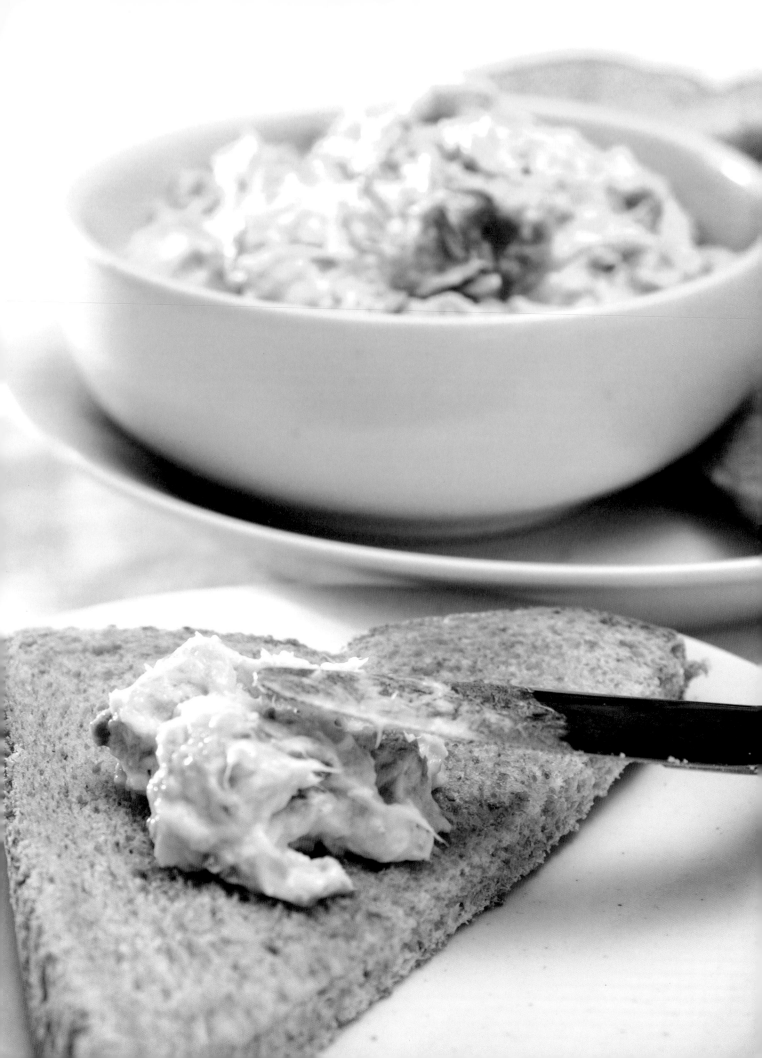

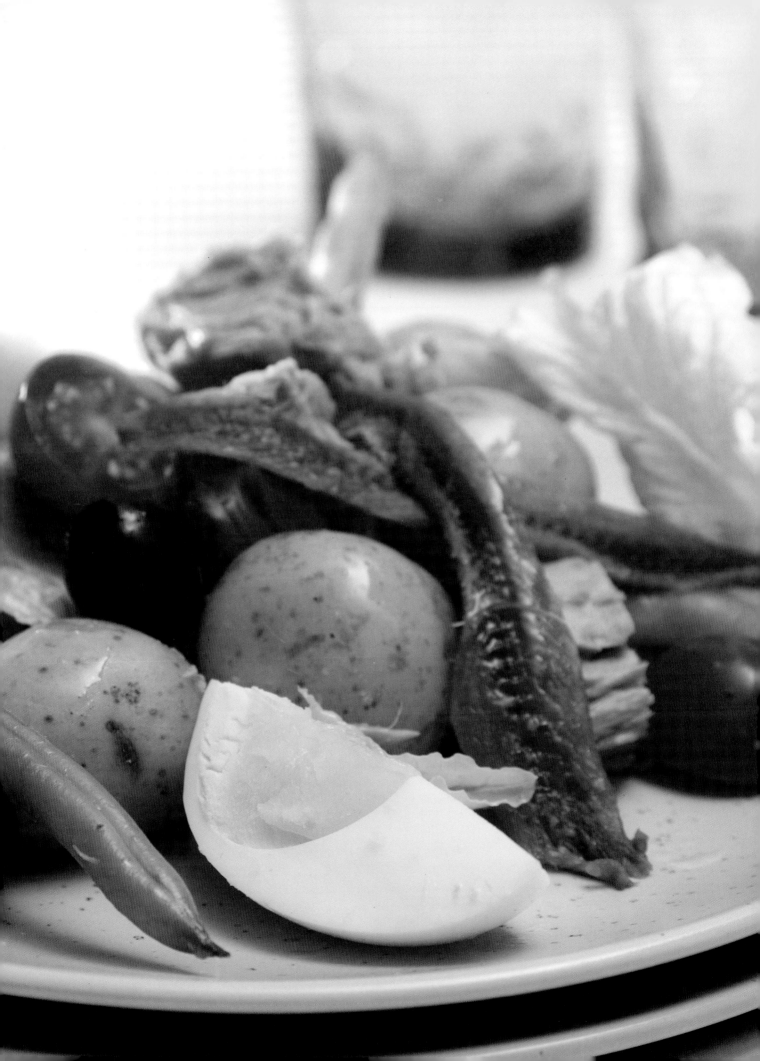

Nicoise Potato Salad

Family Favourite

New potatoes are served with this popular salad to add carbohydrates to the meal. Oily fish such as tuna contain omega 3 oils which are important for a healthy heart.

Ingredients for 2

350g/12oz baby new potatoes
50g/2oz green beans, trimmed
½ head cos lettuce, washed
4 cherry tomatoes, halved
200g/7oz can tuna in spring water, drained
3 tbsp low-fat French dressing
15g/½oz anchovy fillets
1 hard-boiled egg, cut into wedges
4 black olives
freshly ground black pepper

Ingredients for 4

700g/1½lb baby new potatoes
100g/4oz green beans, trimmed
1 head cos lettuce, washed
8 cherry tomatoes, halved
2 x 200g/7oz cans tuna in spring water, drained
6 tbsp low-fat French dressing
25g/1oz anchovy fillets
2 hard-boiled eggs, cut into wedges
8 black olives
freshly ground black pepper

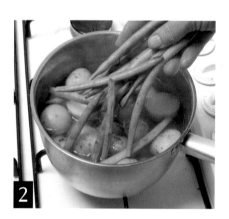

1 Bring a pan of lightly salted water to the boil and cook the potatoes for 12–15 minutes until just tender.

2 Add the beans to the water for the last 3 minutes of the cooking time. Drain and allow to cool.

3 Tear the lettuces into pieces. Toss the potatoes, beans, tomatoes and tuna together. Sprinkle with the dressing, then add the lettuce.

4 Pile on to a serving plate. Drain the anchovies on kitchen paper to remove excess oil.

5 Arrange the eggs, olives and anchovies on top and season lightly with pepper. Serve immediately.

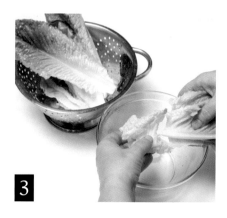

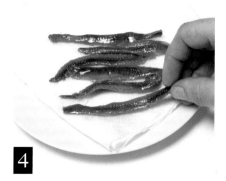

Cheesy Rice Salad

A tasty rice salad that can be eaten at home or transported in an airtight tub and eaten with a small spoon or fork when a packed lunch is required.

Ingredients for 2

50g/2oz reduced-fat Cheddar
  cheese
40g/1½oz cherry tomatoes
40g/1½oz cucumber
200g/7oz cooked brown rice
50g/2oz peeled prawns,
  thawed if frozen
40g/1½oz frozen peas,
  thawed
2 tbsp low-fat vinaigrette
  salad dressing

Ingredients for 4

100g/4oz reduced-fat
  Cheddar cheese
75g/3oz cherry tomatoes
75g/3oz cucumber
400g/14oz cooked brown rice
100g/4oz peeled prawns,
  thawed if frozen
75g/3oz frozen peas, thawed
4 tbsp low-fat vinaigrette
  salad dressing

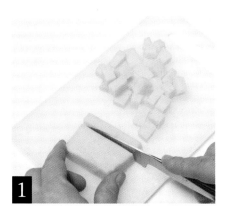

1 Cut the cheese into small cubes.

2 Halve the cherry tomatoes and dice the cucumber.

3 Place the rice in a large bowl, toss with the cheese, prawns, peas, cucumber and tomatoes.

4 Pour the salad dressing over the salad and toss until well coated.

5 Chill until required.

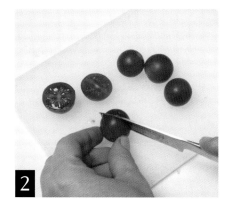

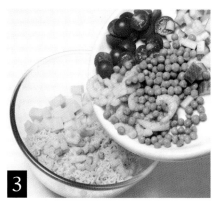

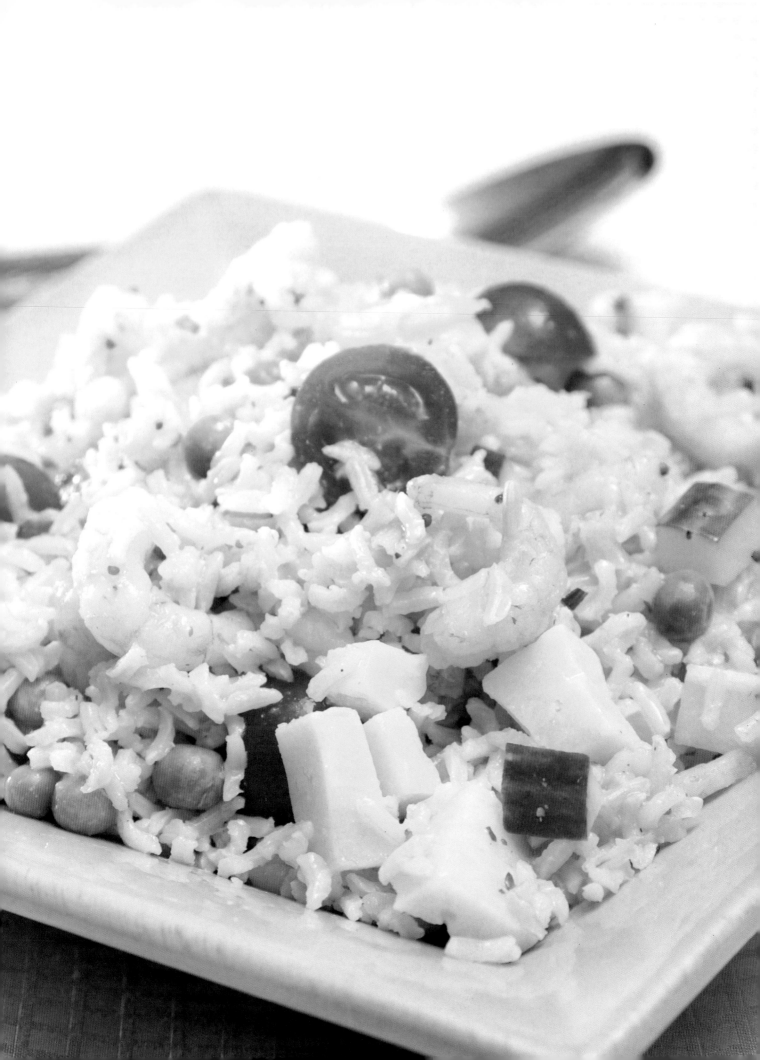

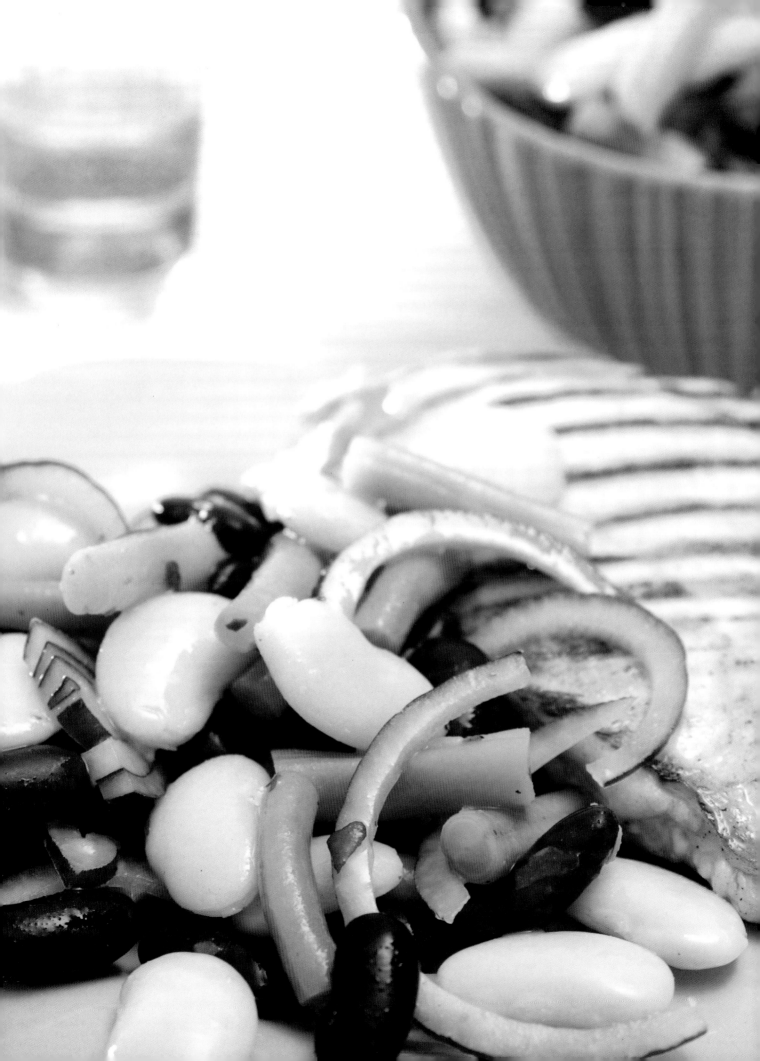

Three Bean Salad with Tuna or Chicken

This delicious salad has lots of soluble fibre, making it an ideal lunch dish for people with diabetes. It can be served at home but is also easily transportable, so it's good for lunch boxes. I like to serve it with chunks of canned tuna (choose tuna packed in spring water), or with a piece of chargrilled chicken.

Ingredients for 2

200g/7oz can red kidney beans, rinsed and drained
200g/7oz can butter beans, rinsed and drained
100g/4oz green beans, trimmed
½ red onion, thinly sliced
3 tbsp low-fat vinaigrette salad dressing
tuna or cooked chicken to serve

Ingredients for 4

400g/14oz can red kidney beans, rinsed and drained
400g/14oz can butter beans, rinsed and drained
200g/7oz green beans, trimmed
1 red onion, thinly sliced
6 tbsp low-fat vinaigrette salad dressing
tuna or cooked chicken to serve

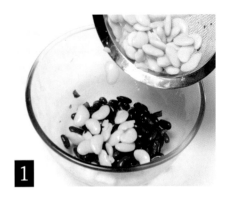

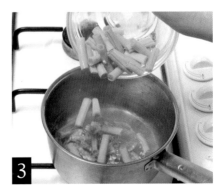

1 Mix the canned beans together in a bowl.

2 Bring a saucepan of water to the boil. Cut the green bean into short lengths.

3 Blanch in the boiling water for 3 minutes, refresh under running cold water and drain again.

4 Add to the canned beans with the red onion.

5 Toss the salad until lightly coated in the dressing.

6 Serve with the tuna or chicken.

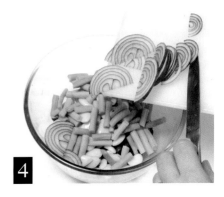

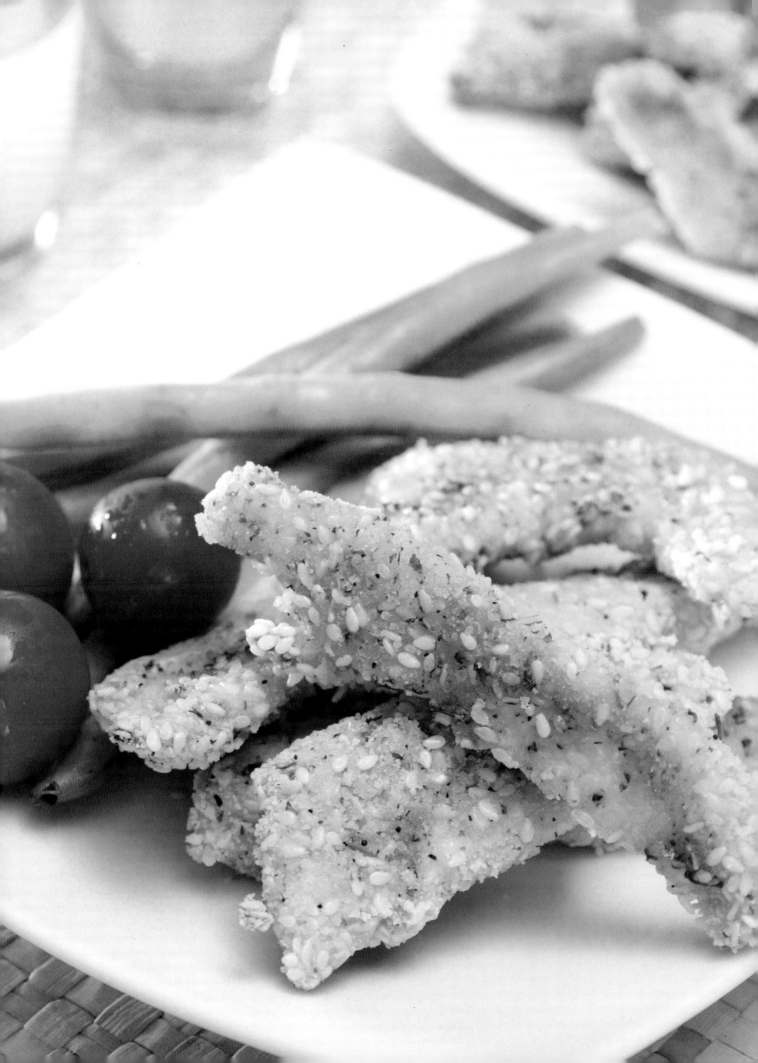

Sesame Chicken Nuggets

Freezer Friendly

This is a very popular recipe in my house, as it is so versatile. Home-made chicken nuggets have much less fat than those from fast-food outlets and taste better too. I often double up quantities so that I can freeze them for a later meal. They can be frozen, cooked, defrosted and eaten cold, or frozen uncooked, defrosted and cooked when required.

Ingredients for 2

- **2 skinless and boneless chicken breasts**
- **salt and freshly ground black pepper**
- **1 small egg**
- **40g/1½oz dried natural or golden breadcrumbs**
- **3 tbsp sesame seeds**
- **½ tsp dried mixed herbs**
- **1 tbsp plain flour**
- **1 tsp sunflower oil**

Ingredients for 4

- **4 skinless and boneless chicken breasts**
- **salt and freshly ground black pepper**
- **1 large egg**
- **75g/3oz dried natural or golden breadcrumbs**
- **6 tbsp sesame seeds**
- **1 tsp dried mixed herbs**
- **2 tbsp plain flour**
- **2 tsp sunflower oil**

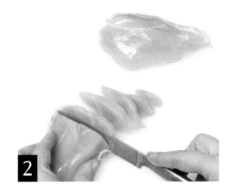

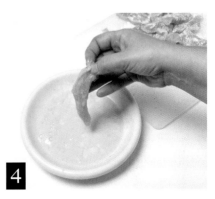

1 Preheat the oven to 200°C/400°F/gas mark 6. Lightly oil a baking sheet.

2 Cut the chicken into strips. Season with salt and pepper.

3 Lightly beat the egg in a bowl. Combine the breadcrumbs, sesame seeds and herbs and spread out on a plate.

4 Dust the chicken strips with flour, then dip in the egg.

5 Next coat them with the sesame seed mixture.

6 Lay in a single layer on the sheet.

7 Drizzle the oil over the nuggets and bake in the centre of the oven for 15 minutes or until crisp and golden.

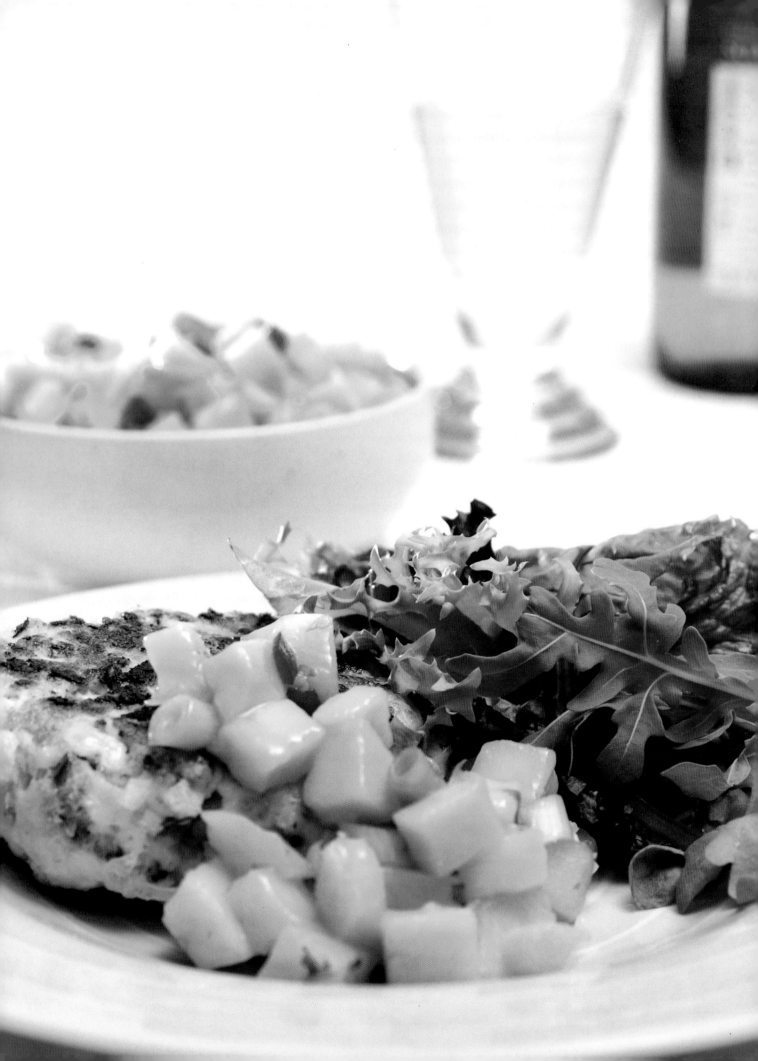

Chicken Burger with Mango Salsa

Family Favourite

Poultry is a low-fat meat. You can use ready-minced chicken, but I prefer to buy chicken breasts and mince it myself in a food processor. If you are making this for two, the remaining salsa can be served with grilled meat or fish at another meal. Serve the burgers with bread or potatoes for a balanced meal.

Ingredients for 2

- 225g/8oz chicken meat, minced
- 2 spring onions, finely chopped
- 15g/½oz fresh wholemeal breadcrumbs
- 1 tbsp fresh coriander, chopped

Ingredients for 4

- 450g/1lb chicken meat, minced
- 4 spring onions, finely chopped
- 25g/1oz fresh wholemeal breadcrumbs
- 2 tbsp fresh coriander, chopped

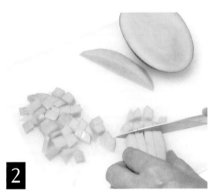

Mango salsa:

- 1 mango
- 4 spring onions, sliced
- 2 tbsp lemon juice
- 2 tbsp coriander, chopped
- 1 red or green chilli, seeded and chopped (optional)

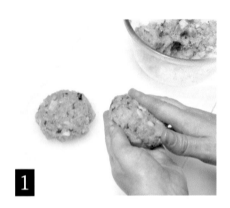

1 Mix together the chicken, onion, breadcrumbs and coriander until well combined. Shape into 4 (8) burgers.

2 Peel, and stone the mango and cut the flesh into small dice.

3 Place in a bowl with the remaining salsa ingredients and mix well. Chill until required.

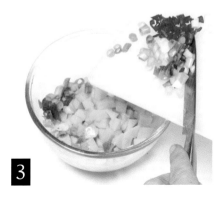

4 Cook the burgers under a preheated grill for 4–5 minutes each side or until cooked through.

5 Serve the burgers with the mango salsa.

Orange Glazed Chicken Drumsticks

Family Favourite

I love recipes that can be eaten hot or cold, as they are so versatile. When the kids are home from school I serve this with new potatoes and fresh vegetables. As a term-time lunch they often have these cold in their lunch boxes with carrot sticks and cucumber to nibble, and a chunk of wholemeal bread.

Ingredients for 2

4 chicken drumsticks
grated zest and juice ½
   orange
pinch of ground ginger
2 tbsp clear honey
½ tsp wholegrain mustard

Ingredients for 4

8 chicken drumsticks
grated zest and juice 1
   orange
¼ tsp ground ginger
4 tbsp clear honey
1 tsp wholegrain mustard

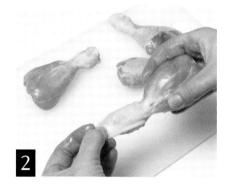

1 Preheat the oven to 180°C/350°F/gas mark 4. Lightly grease a baking sheet.

2 Skin the chicken (most of the fat is just under the skin).

3 Combine the orange zest, juice, ginger, honey and mustard. Brush over the chicken.

4 Place on the baking sheet and bake for 15 minutes. Brush with the remaining glaze and return to the oven. Bake for a further 10 minutes or until the juices run clear.

5 Serve hot or cold.

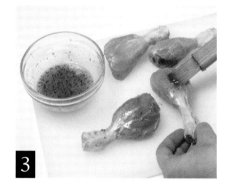

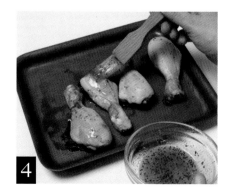

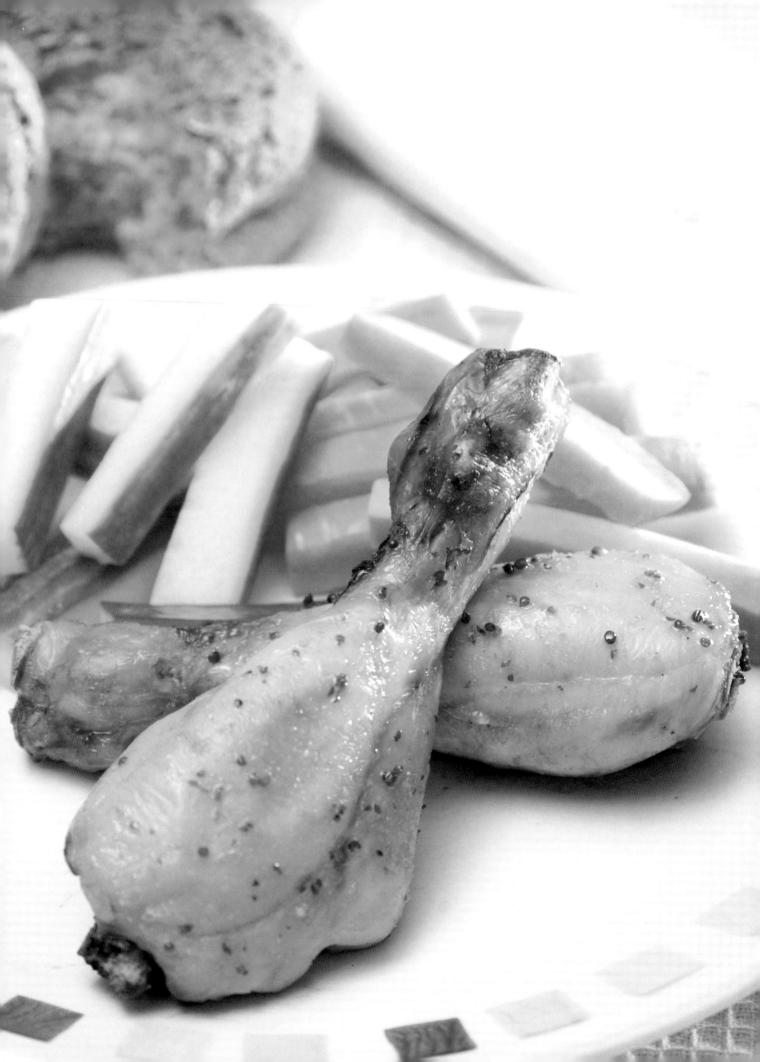

Meat Loaf

The addition of lentils to the meat loaf adds valuable soluble fibre and reduces the amount of meat and, therefore, the amount of saturated fat. Serve with salad and new potatoes or bread.

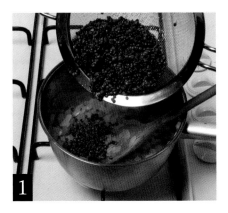

Ingredients for 4

1 tsp olive oil
1 small carrot, chopped
1 stick celery, chopped
1 small onion, chopped
60g/2½oz green lentils
200g/7oz can chopped
    tomatoes
150ml/¼pt hot beef stock
175g/6oz lean mince beef
50g/2oz wholemeal
    breadcrumbs
1 tsp dried mixed herbs
1 tbsp tomato purée
1 egg, beaten
salt and freshly ground
    black pepper

Ingredients for 8

2 tsp olive oil
1 large carrot, chopped
2 sticks celery, chopped
1 onion, chopped
150g/5oz green lentils
400g/14oz can chopped
    tomatoes
300ml/½pt hot beef stock
350g/12oz lean mince beef
100g/4oz wholemeal
    breadcrumbs
2 tsp dried mixed herbs
2 tbsp tomato purée
2 eggs, beaten
salt and freshly ground
    black pepper

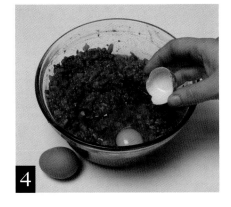

1 Heat the oil in a saucepan and sauté the carrot, celery and onion for 5 minutes until softened. Add the lentils, tomatoes and stock and bring to the boil.

2 Reduce the heat, cover and simmer for 20–25 minutes until the liquid has been absorbed and the lentils are tender.

3 Lightly grease a 450g/1lb (900g/2lb) loaf tin. Preheat the oven to 180°C/350°F/gas mark 4.

4 Add all the remaining ingredients to the lentils and mix well.

5 Pile into the loaf tin and press down well.

6 Cover with foil and bake for 30 (45) minutes. Remove the foil and return to the oven for 15 minutes.

7 Allow to stand in the tin for 15 minutes, before turning out. Delicious served hot or cold.

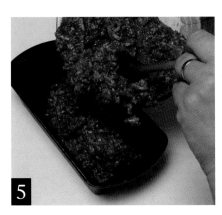

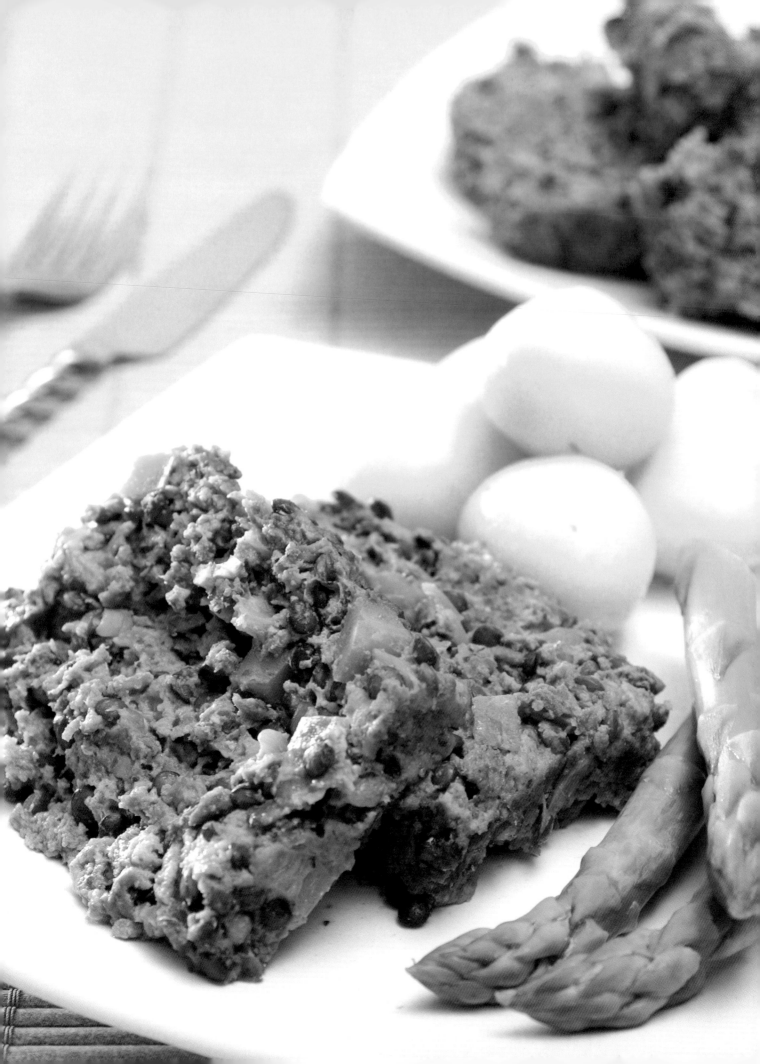

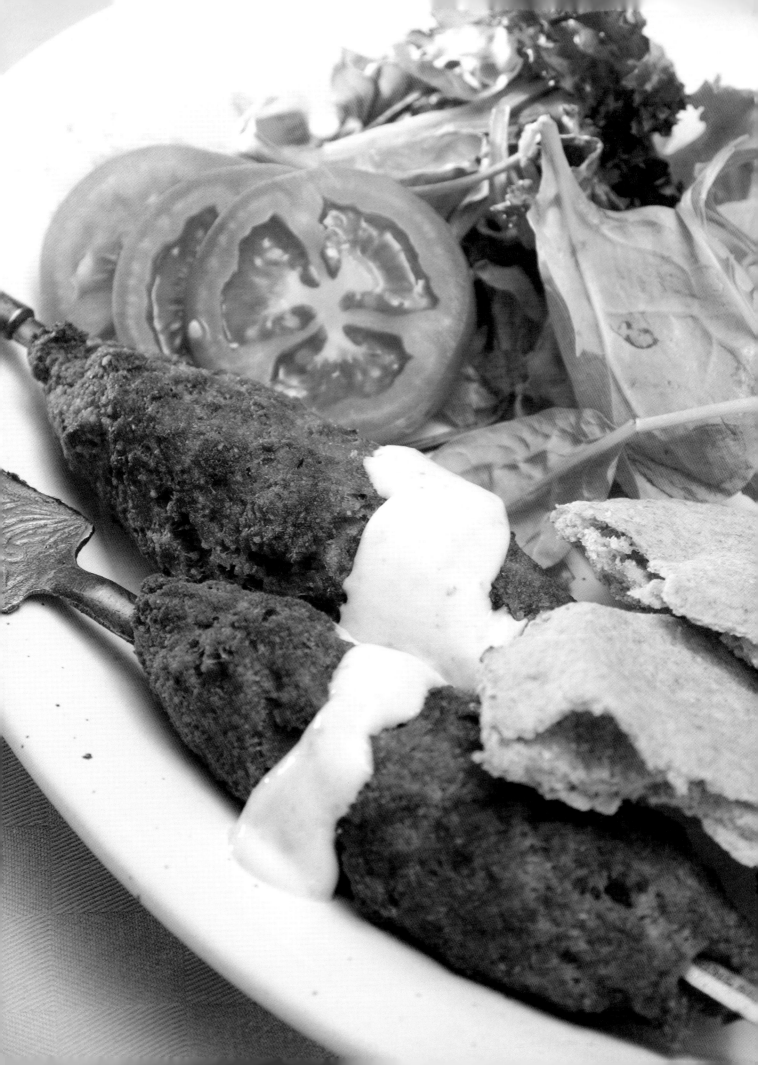

Lamb Kofte

This is an economical dish which tastes fantastic. Couscous stretches the meat so that it goes further, and it also provides soluble fibre. You can vary the spices added to the meat mixture to ring the changes. Also try serving with a spicy tomato salsa. Accompany with a mixed salad and pitta bread.

Ingredients for 2

40g/1½oz couscous
150ml/¼pt boiling water
½ tsp chilli powder
¼ tsp each ground cinnamon, coriander and cumin
200g/7oz lean minced lamb
½ small onion, chopped
salt and freshly ground black pepper
½ tsp concentrated mint sauce
75ml/2½fl oz reduced-fat Greek-style yoghurt
pinch of sugar

Ingredients for 4

75g/3oz couscous
300ml/½pt boiling water
1 tsp chilli powder
½ tsp each ground cinnamon, coriander and cumin
400g/14oz lean minced lamb
1 small onion, chopped
salt and freshly ground black pepper
1 tsp concentrated mint sauce
150ml/¼pt reduced-fat Greek-style yoghurt
pinch of sugar

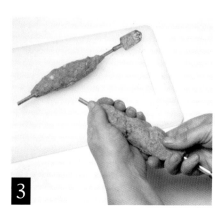

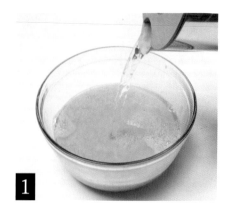

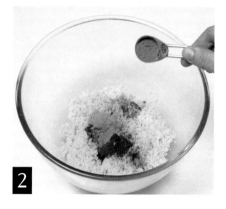

1 Place the couscous in a bowl and pour the boiling water over it. Allow to stand for about 20 minutes. Drain and squeeze out as much moisture as you can. Allow to cool.

2 Sprinkle the spices over the couscous and mix in with a fork. Add the lamb and onion, season well and knead together until well combined.

3 Divide the mixture into 4 (8) and shape into tapered sausage shape around skewers.

4 Cook under a hot grill for 10–15 minutes, turning frequently until cooked through.

5 Meanwhile, squeeze out the excess vinegar from the mint sauce and stir the mint into the yoghurt with the sugar.

6 Serve the kebabs with the mint sauce spooned over.

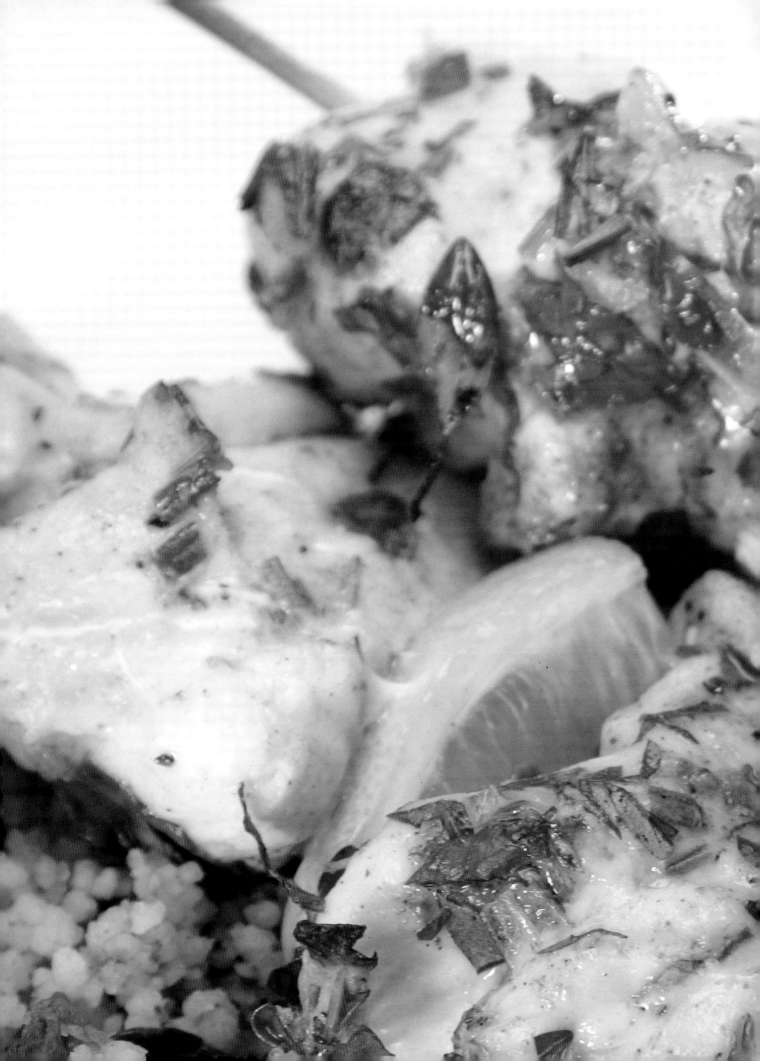

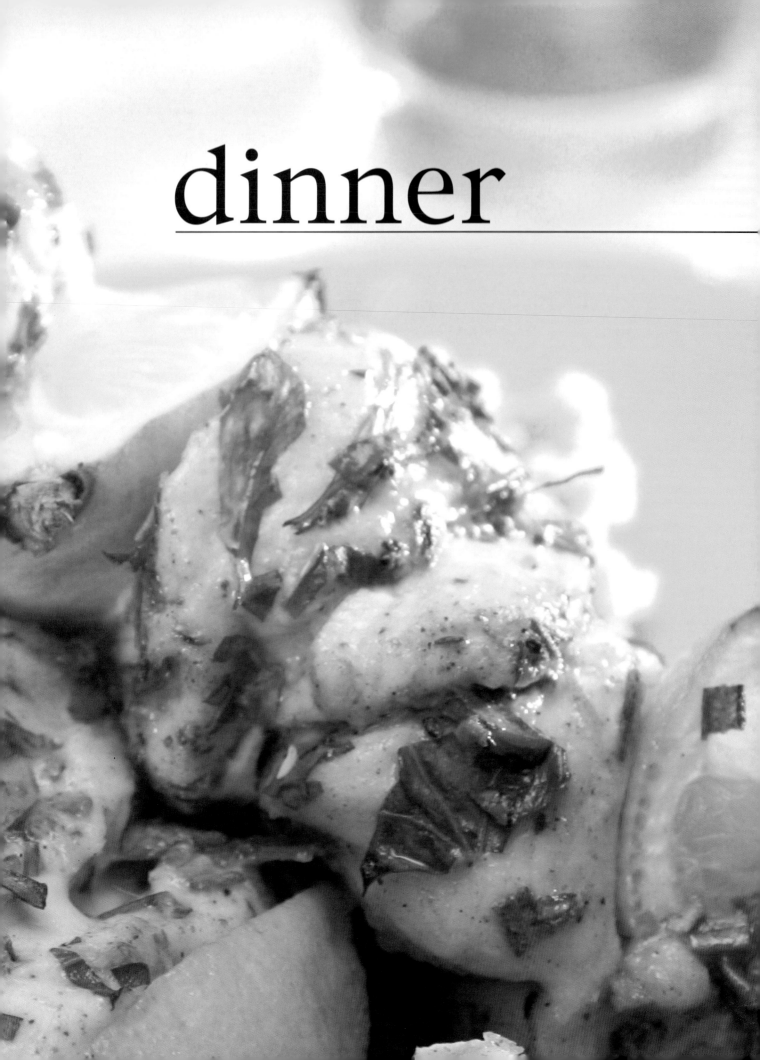

dinner

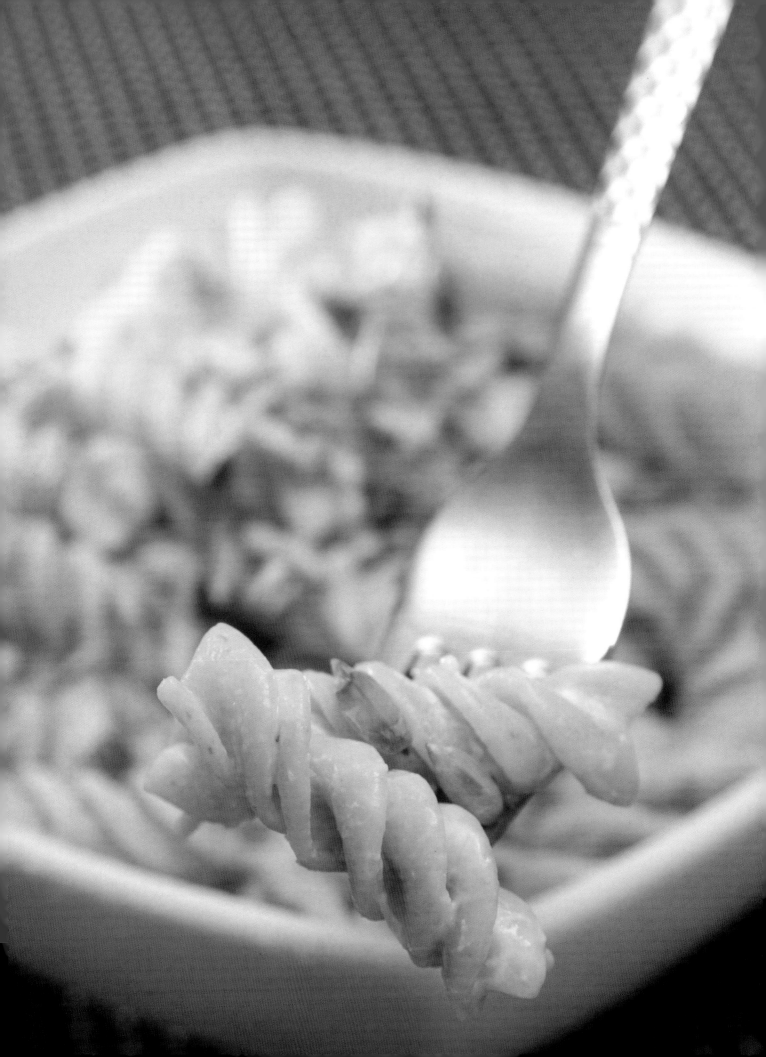

Penne with Herb & Garlic Sauce

Quick and easy

Use wholemeal penne if you can find them. The garlicky sauce tastes so good you will not realise that this is a low-fat creamy sauce. Serve with a mixed salad.

Ingredients for 2

175g/6oz penne
1 tbsp sunflower seeds
1 tsp sunflower oil
½ small onion, chopped
75g/3oz low-fat garlic and
   herb soft cheese
4 tbsp skimmed or semi-
   skimmed milk
salt and freshly ground
   black pepper

Ingredients for 4

350g/12oz penne
2 tbsp sunflower seeds
1 tsp sunflower oil
1 small onion, chopped
150g/5oz low-fat garlic and
   herb soft cheese
125ml/4fl oz skimmed or
   semi-skimmed milk
salt and freshly ground
   black pepper

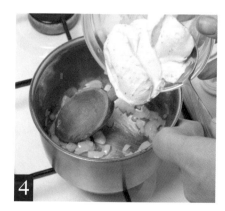

1 Cook the pasta in plenty of lightly salted boiling water for 10–12 minutes, or as directed on the packet.

2 Meanwhile place the sunflower seeds in a heavy based non-stick frying pan and cook over a medium heat until browned, shaking the pan a few times as they cook. Then set aside.

3 In a small pan heat the oil and fry the onion for 1–2 minutes until softened.

4 Add the cheese and milk and heat gently, stirring until well combined.

5 Drain the pasta. Stir in the cheese sauce.

6 Serve immediately, sprinkled with the sunflower seeds.

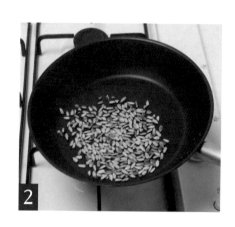

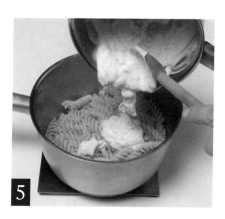

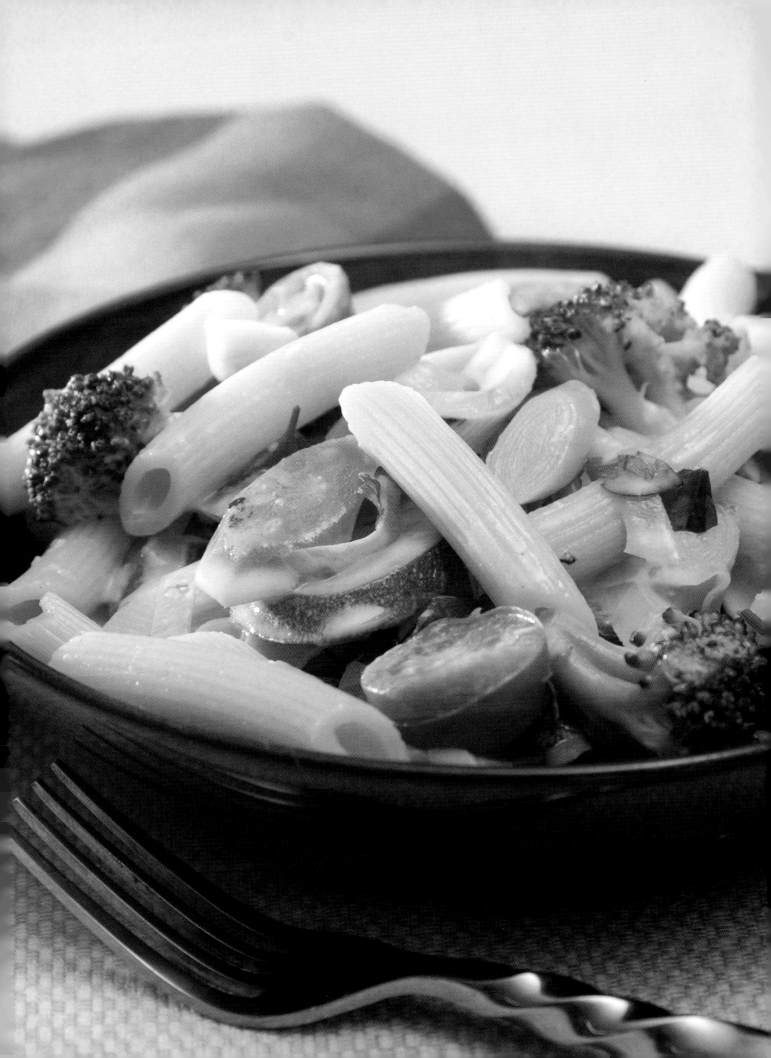

Pasta Primavera

vegetarian

Lots of fresh vegetables in a light creamy sauce make this a great midweek meal. The vegetables will count as two portions of your five-a-day.

Ingredients for 2

175g/6oz wholemeal pasta
100g/4oz broccoli
2 tsp olive oil
½ leek, sliced
½ head fennel, trimmed and sliced
1 small courgette, trimmed and sliced
1 carrot, sliced
salt and freshly ground black pepper
2 tbsp fresh parsley, coarsely chopped
75g/3oz cherry tomatoes, halved
100g/4oz low-fat crème fraîche
25g/1oz Parmesan cheese, grated

Ingredients for 4

350g/12oz wholemeal pasta
225g/8oz broccoli
4 tsp olive oil
1 leek, sliced
1 head fennel, trimmed and sliced
1 courgette, trimmed and sliced
2 carrots, sliced
salt and freshly ground black pepper
4 tbsp fresh parsley, coarsely chopped
175g/6oz cherry tomatoes, halved
200g/7oz low-fat crème fraîche
50g/2oz Parmesan cheese, grated

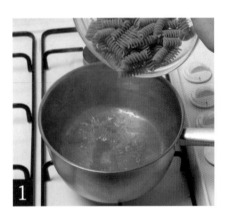

1 Cook the pasta in plenty of lightly salted boiling water for 10 minutes, or as directed on the packet. Drain.

2 Meanwhile, cut the broccoli into small florets. Cut away the tough bottom part of the stalk and thinly slice the stem.

3 Heat the oil in a large non-stick frying pan over a medium heat. Add the broccoli stems, leek and fennel and sauté gently for 2 minutes.

4 Add the broccoli florets, courgettes and carrot. Add a few tablespoons of water to the pan so that the vegetables begin to steam. Cook for 3–5 minutes or until just tender but still with a little bit of bite, adding a little more water if required. Season with a little salt and pepper.

5 Stir the parsley, tomatoes, crème fraîche and Parmesan into the pan and cook, stirring constantly for 2 minutes. Remove from the heat. Add to the pasta and toss to combine.

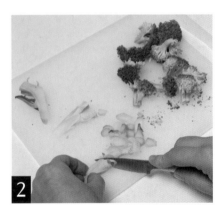

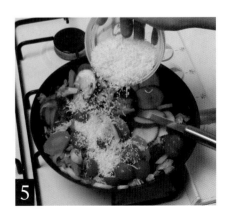

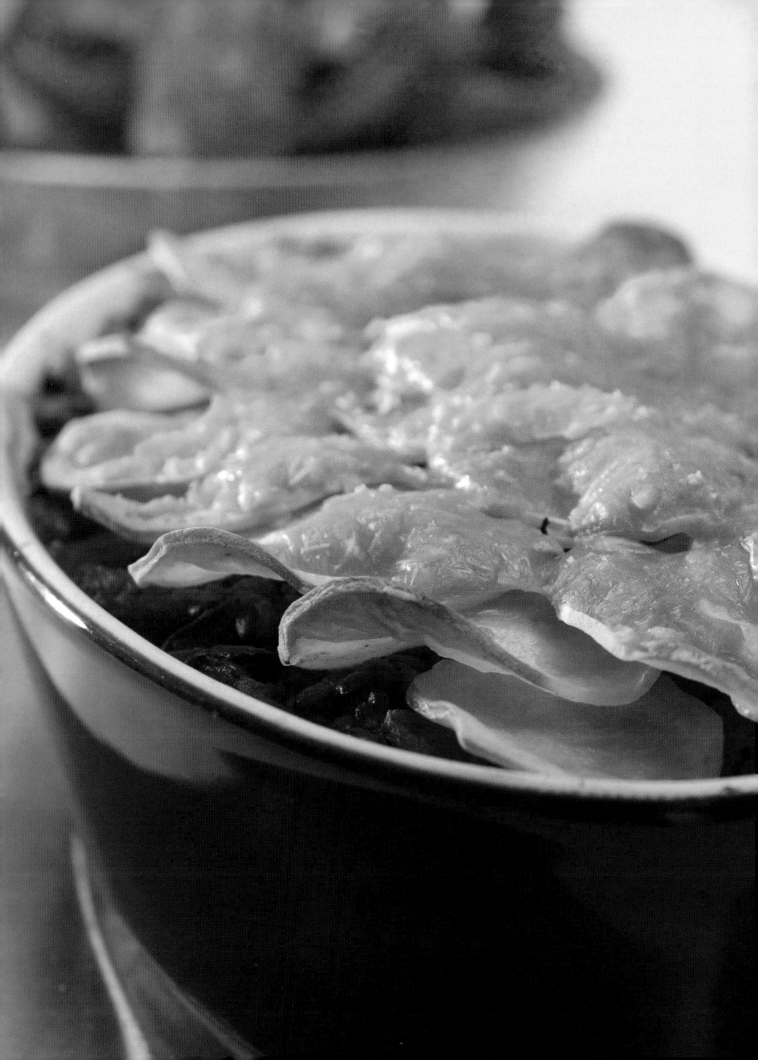

Lentil Hot Pot

Lentils are convenient because they do not need soaking. Puy lentils are reputed to have the best flavour, but I find this robustly flavoured hotpot is fine made with any green lentils (lentils vertes). Serve with a fresh green vegetable and some crusty bread.

Ingredients for 2

1 tsp sunflower oil
1 onion, sliced
75g/3oz green lentils, rinsed
200g/7oz can chopped
    tomatoes
1 tsp mixed dried herbs
salt and freshly ground
    black pepper
350g/12oz potatoes, sliced
100ml/3½fl oz vegetable
    stock
25g/1oz reduced-fat red
    Leicester cheese

Ingredients for 4

2 tsp sunflower oil
2 onions, sliced
150g/5oz green lentils, rinsed
400g/14oz can chopped
    tomatoes
2 tsp mixed dried herbs
salt and freshly ground
    black pepper
700g/1½lb potatoes, sliced
200ml/7fl oz vegetable stock
50g/2oz reduced-fat red
    Leicester cheese

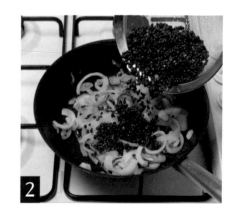

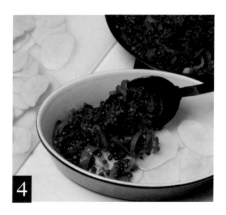

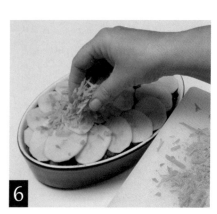

1 Heat the oil in a non-stick frying pan and fry the onions for 5 minutes until beginning to soften.

2 Stir in the lentils, chopped tomatoes, 150ml/¼pt (300ml/½pt) water and herbs and bring to the boil. Reduce the heat and simmer gently for 20–30 minutes until lentils are soft but still hold their shape. Season to taste

3 Preheat the oven to 180°C/350°F/gas mark 4.

4 Place a layer of potatoes in the bottom of a deep ovenproof dish. Spoon about one-quarter of the lentil mixture on top.

5 Repeat the layers until all the lentil mixture has been used and finish with a layer of potato. Carefully pour the stock over the potatoes.

6 Sprinkle the cheese over the top.

7 Bake in the centre of the oven for 50–60 minutes. Cover with foil if the top begins to brown too much.

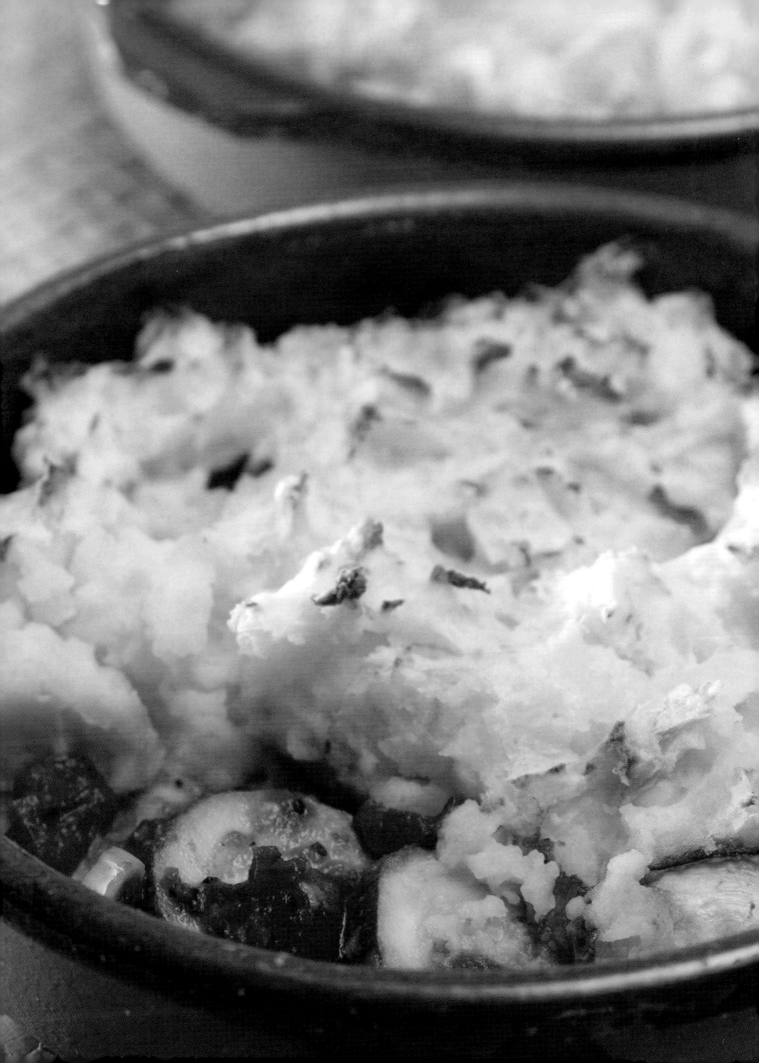

Courgette & Tomato Bake

vegetarian

Adding celeriac to the potato gives this vegetarian version of shepherd's pie much more flavour. This is a meal in itself, or it can be served with a fresh green vegetable.

Ingredients for 2

1 tsp olive oil
1 leek, sliced
250g/9oz courgettes, sliced
1 clove garlic, chopped
200g/7oz can chopped
    tomatoes with herbs
2 tsp tomato purée
350g/12oz potatoes, peeled
    and cut into cubes
175g/6oz celeriac, peeled and
    cut into cubes
2 tbsp skimmed or
    semi-skimmed milk
salt and freshly ground
    black pepper

Ingredients for 4

2 tsp olive oil
2 leeks, sliced
500g/1lb 2oz courgettes,
    sliced
2 cloves garlic, chopped
400g/14oz can chopped
    tomatoes with herbs
1 tbsp tomato purée
700g/1½lb potatoes, peeled
    and cut into cubes
350g/12oz celeriac, peeled
    and cut into cubes
4 tbsp skimmed or
    semi-skimmed milk
salt and freshly ground
    black pepper

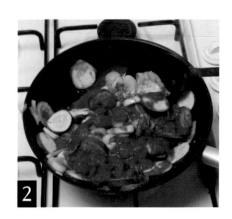

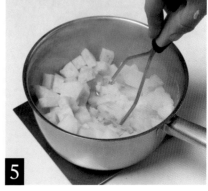

1 Heat the oil in a non-stick frying pan and sauté the leeks and courgettes for 3–4 minutes until beginning to soften. Add the garlic and sauté for 1 minute.

2 Stir in the tomatoes and tomato purée and bring to the boil, Simmer for 5 minutes and season to taste.

3 Pour into a shallow ovenproof dish. Preheat the oven to 200°C/400°F/gas mark 6.

4 Cook the potatoes and celeriac in lightly salted boiling water for 10–15 minutes until just tender.

5 Drain well. Add the milk, season with salt and pepper, and mash until smooth.

6 Spread over the tomato and courgette mixture and bake for 35–40 minutes until golden.

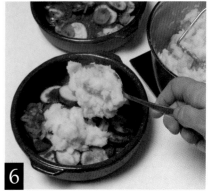

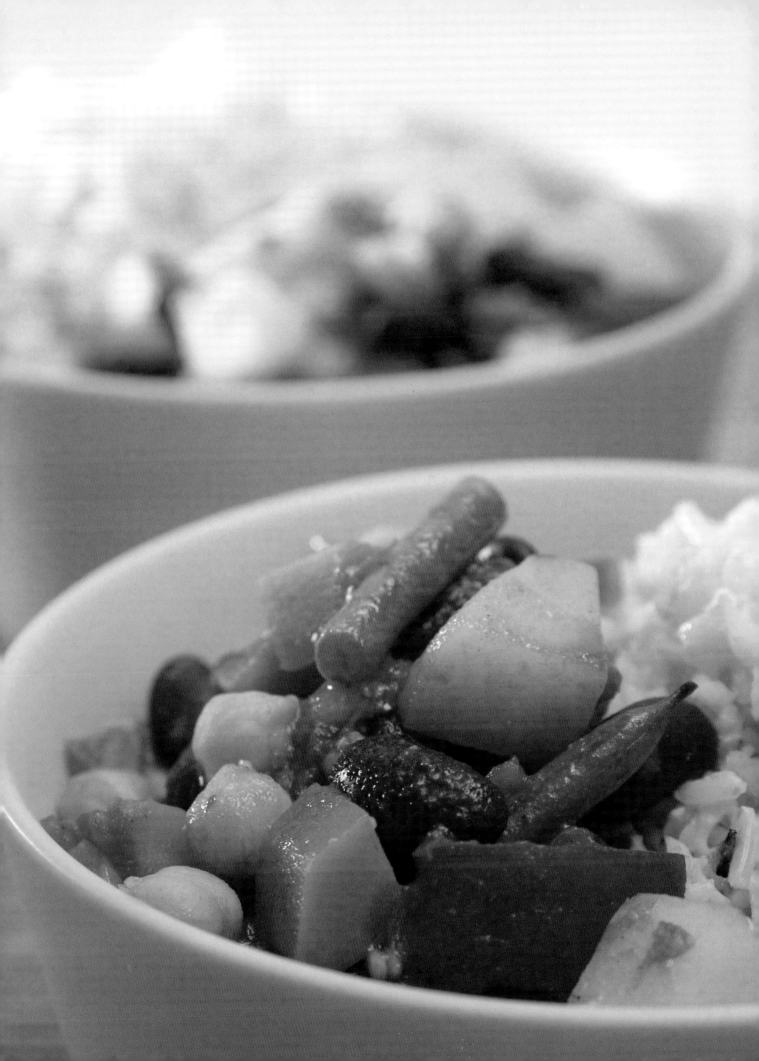

Vegetable Chilli

vegetarian

Chilli is a popular dish and with fresh vegetables and beans it is a good choice for people with diabetes. Often made with meat, this version is vegetarian and lower in fat than a meaty chilli con carne. Serve with brown rice

Ingredients for 2

1 tsp sunflower oil
1 small onion, chopped
1 clove garlic, chopped
100g/4oz waxy potatoes, cut into large dice
1 large carrot, peeled and diced
50g/2oz green beans, trimmed and cut into 2cm/1in lengths
½ red pepper, seeded and cut into chunks
1 tsp chilli purée, or extra to taste
75ml/2½fl oz vegetable stock
200g/7oz can chopped tomatoes
200g/7oz can red kidney beans, rinsed and drained
200g/7oz can chick peas, rinsed and drained
brown rice to serve

Ingredients for 4

2 tsp sunflower oil
1 large onion, chopped
1 clove garlic, chopped
225g/8oz waxy potatoes, cut into large dice
2 large carrots, peeled and diced
100g/4oz green beans, trimmed and cut into 2cm/1in lengths
1 red pepper, seeded and cut into chunks
2 tsp chilli purée, or extra to taste
150ml/¼pt vegetable stock
400g/14oz can chopped tomatoes
400g/14oz can red kidney beans, rinsed and drained
400g/14oz can chick peas, rinsed and drained
brown rice to serve

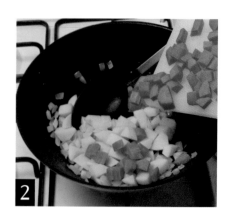

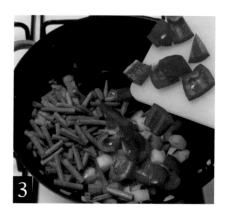

1 Heat the oil in a large non-stick frying pan and fry the onion and garlic for 2–3 minutes until beginning to soften.

2 Add the potatoes and the carrot to the pan and fry for 5 minutes until the vegetables begin to colour.

3 Add the green beans and peppers, and cook for a further 5 minutes.

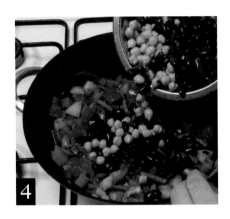

4 Stir in the chilli purée, stock, chopped tomatoes, red kidney beans and chick peas.

5 Bring to the boil, then reduce the heat and simmer for 35–40 minutes until all the vegetables are tender and the flavours are well combined. Serve with brown rice.

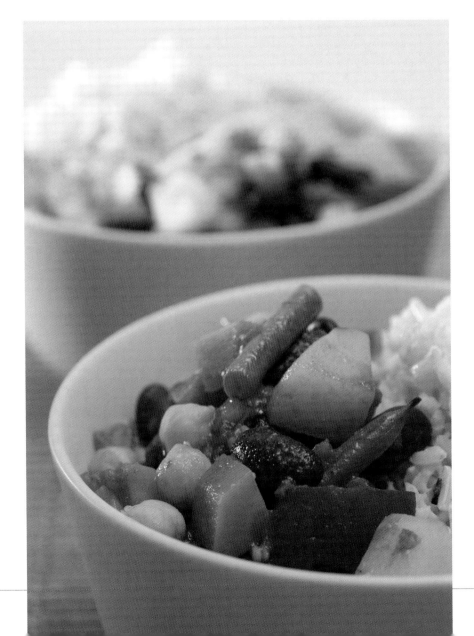

Moroccan Chicken Kebabs

Easy Entertaining

Raz-el hanout is an aromatic, slightly floral blend of spices from Morocco. If you cannot find it, choose another couscous spice blend instead.

Ingredients for 2

250g/9oz skinned and boned chicken breasts
½ lemon
2 tsp fresh parsley, chopped
2 tsp fresh rosemary, chopped
1 tsp fresh thyme leaves
1 clove garlic, crushed
½ tsp raz-el hanout
1 tsp olive oil

Couscous:

75g/3oz couscous
25g/1oz sultanas
1-2 tsp raz-el hanout

Ingredients for 4

500g/1lb 2oz skinned and boned chicken breasts
1 lemon
4 tsp fresh parsley, chopped
4 tsp fresh rosemary, chopped
2 tsp fresh thyme leaves
2 cloves garlic, crushed
1 tsp raz-el hanout
2 tsp olive oil

Couscous:

175g/6oz couscous
50g/2oz sultanas
1 tbsp raz-el hanout

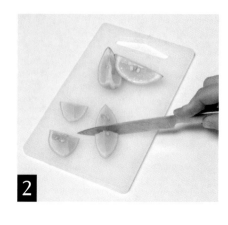

1 Cut the chicken into cubes.

2 Using half of the lemon, cut it into wedges, then cut the wedges in half. Set aside.

3 Grate the zest and squeeze the juice from the remaining lemon. Mix with the herbs, garlic, spice and olive oil in a shallow non-metallic dish.

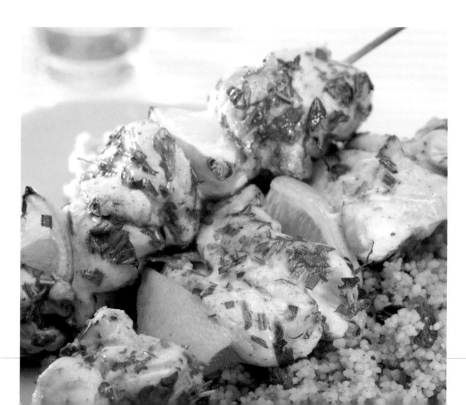

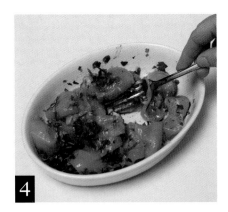

4

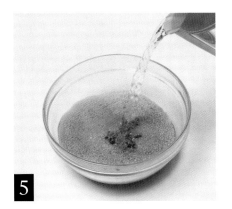

5

4 Add the chicken and toss in the marinade. Allow to marinate for at least 1 hour or up to 24 hours in the refrigerator.

5 To make the couscous, place it in a bowl with the sultanas and spices. Add boiling water until it covers the couscous by about 1cm/½in. Allow to stand for 30 minutes and then drain well. Fluff with a fork.

6 Meanwhile thread the chicken and reserved lemon pieces on to skewers.

7 Cook the chicken under a preheated grill for 10–15 minutes, turning frequently. Serve with the couscous

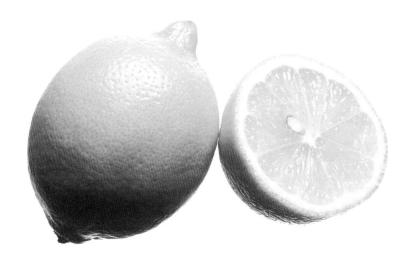

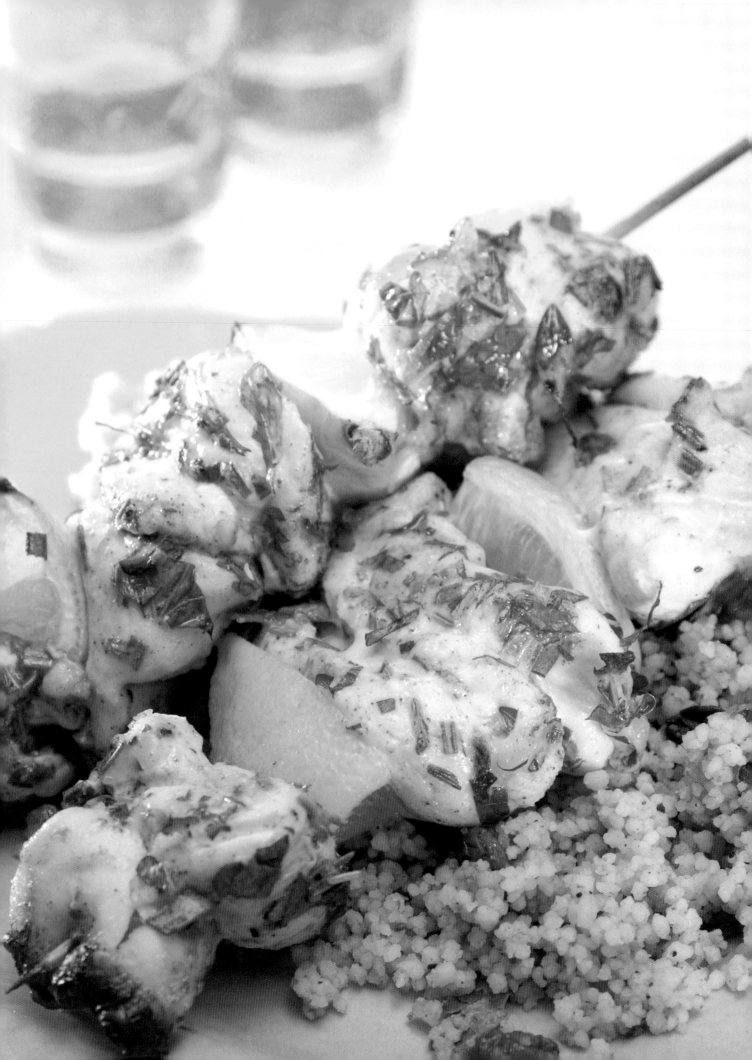

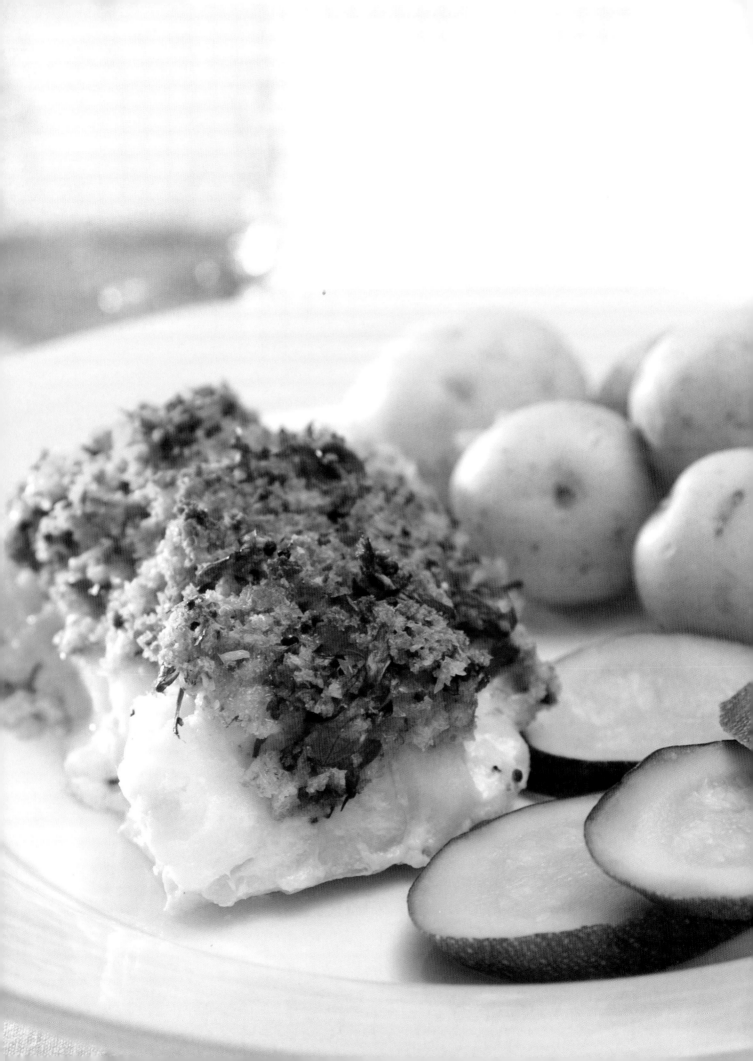

Cod with a Herb & Mustard Crust

Quick and easy

This simple dish is ideal for a midweek meal when you do not want to spend too much time in the kitchen. Serve with new potatoes and fresh vegetables. I keep fresh breadcrumbs in the freezer as they can be used from frozen. This dish can also be made with salmon.

Ingredients for 2

2 x 150g/5oz cod fillets
salt and freshly ground
  black pepper
25g/1oz reduced-fat mature
  Cheddar, finely grated
50g/2oz fresh wholemeal
  breadcrumbs
2 tbsp flat leaf parsley,
  chopped
1-2 tsp wholegrain
  mustard
1 tsp olive oil
2 tbsp water

Ingredients for 4

4 x 150g/5oz cod fillets
salt and freshly ground
  black pepper
50g/2oz reduced-fat mature
  Cheddar, finely grated
100g/4oz fresh wholemeal
  breadcrumbs
4 tbsp flat leaf parsley,
  chopped
1 tbsp wholegrain mustard
2 tsp olive oil
4 tbsp water

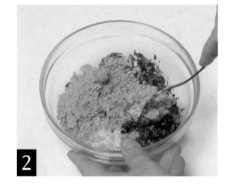

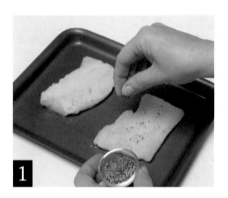

1 Preheat the oven to 200°C/400°F/gas mark 6. Season the cod with salt and pepper.

2 Mix together the cheese, breadcrumbs, parsley, mustard, oil and just enough water to make the mixture begin to bind together.

3 Place the cod in a shallow roasting tin and top with the breadcrumb mixture.

4 Bake for 10–15 minutes until the cod is just flaking and the topping is golden.

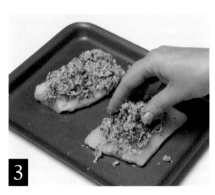

Trout with Nutty Rice Stuffing

This is a great dish for using up left-over cooked rice. Trout is an oily fish that contains important omega 3 oils which are needed for a healthy heart. Try to eat oily fish at least once a week. Serve with some crusty brown bread for carbohydrate and some fresh vegetables.

Ingredients for 2

2 trout, cleaned
salt and freshly ground
 black pepper
1 tsp sunflower oil
½ small onion, chopped
25g/1oz toasted hazelnuts,
 chopped
grated zest ½ orange
1 tbsp orange juice
100g/4oz cooked brown rice
a little beaten egg
orange wedges to serve

Ingredients for 4

4 trout, cleaned
salt and freshly ground
 black pepper
2 tsp sunflower oil
1 small onion, chopped
50g/2oz toasted hazelnuts,
 chopped
grated zest 1 orange
2 tbsp orange juice
225g/8oz cooked brown rice
1 small egg lightly beaten
orange wedges to serve

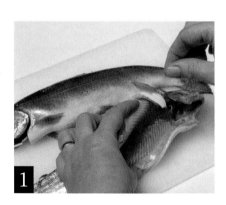

1 Preheat the oven to 180°C/350°F/gas mark 4.

2 Season the cavity of the fish with salt and pepper.

3 Heat the oil in a non-stick frying pan and fry the onion until softened. Remove from the heat.

4 Mix with the hazelnuts, orange zest, juice, rice and enough egg to just bring the mixture together.

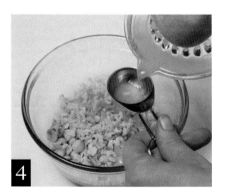

5 Divide the filling between the trout and place in an ovenproof dish.

6 Bake for 20–25 minutes until cooked. Garnish with orange wedges for squeezing.

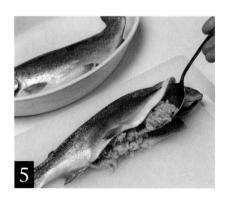

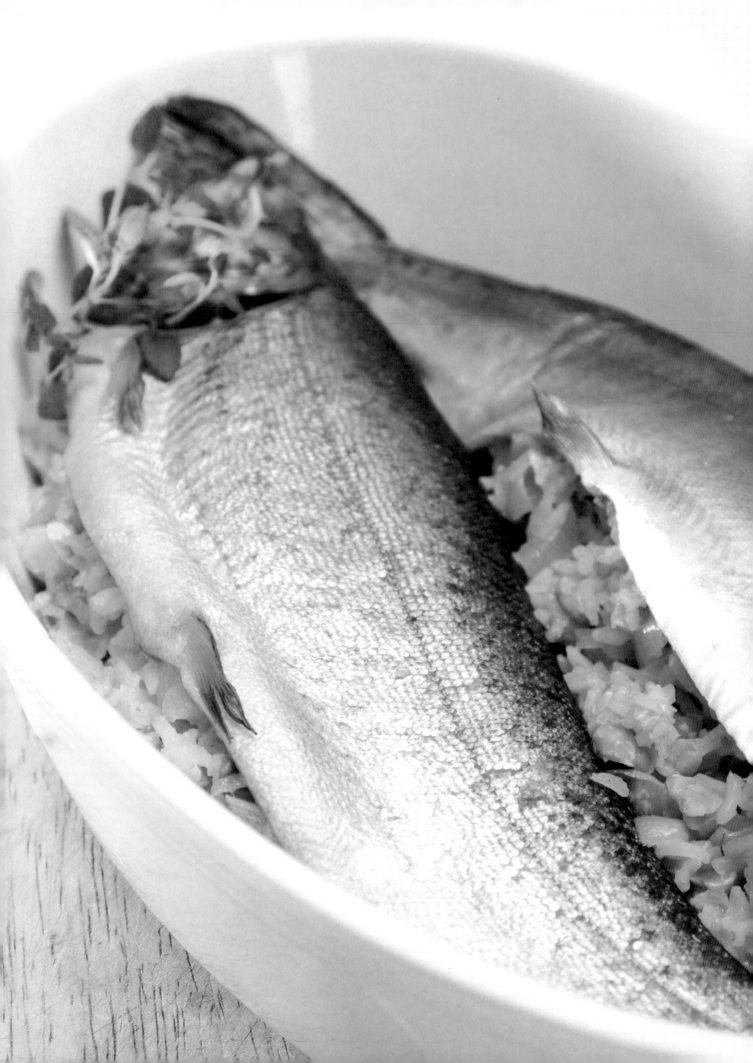

Salmon Steaks with Oriental Coleslaw

Don't be put off by the long list of ingredients – this is a simple and very tasty summer salad to put together. If you have one, use a food processor to prepare, shred and grate the vegetables. I like to serve the coleslaw with salmon, but it also goes well with chicken.

Ingredients for 2

2 salmon steaks

Coleslaw:

½ diakon/mooli radish
1 small carrot
150g/5oz Chinese leaves
100g/4oz red cabbage
½ small onion, sliced
25g/1oz mangetout, sliced
½ tsp sesame seeds

Dressing:

1 tsp grated root ginger
pinch of caster sugar
2 tbsp rice wine or dry sherry
1 tbsp rice or white wine vinegar
1 tsp sunflower oil
2 tsp soy sauce
½ tsp sesame oil

Ingredients for 4

4 salmon steaks

Coleslaw:

1 diakon/mooli radish
1 small carrot
300g/10½oz Chinese leaves
200g/7oz red cabbage
1 small onion, sliced
50g/2oz mangetout, sliced
1 tsp sesame seeds

Dressing:

2 tsp root ginger, grated
½ tsp caster sugar
4 tbsp rice wine or dry sherry
2 tbsp rice or white wine vinegar
2 tsp sunflower oil
1 tbsp soy sauce
1 tsp sesame oil

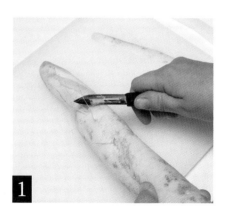

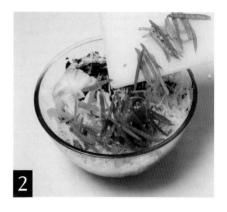

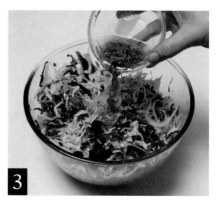

1 Peel and coarsely grate the diakon/mooli and carrots. Shred the Chinese leaves and cabbage.

2 Place all the ingredients for the salad, except the sesame seeds, in a large bowl and toss to combine.

3 Mix together all the ingredients for the dressing and pour over the vegetables. Toss well. Sprinkle over the sesame seeds.

4 Cook the salmon under a preheated grill or on a hot griddle pan for 3–4 minutes each side, until they are cooked through. Serve with the coleslaw and some bread.

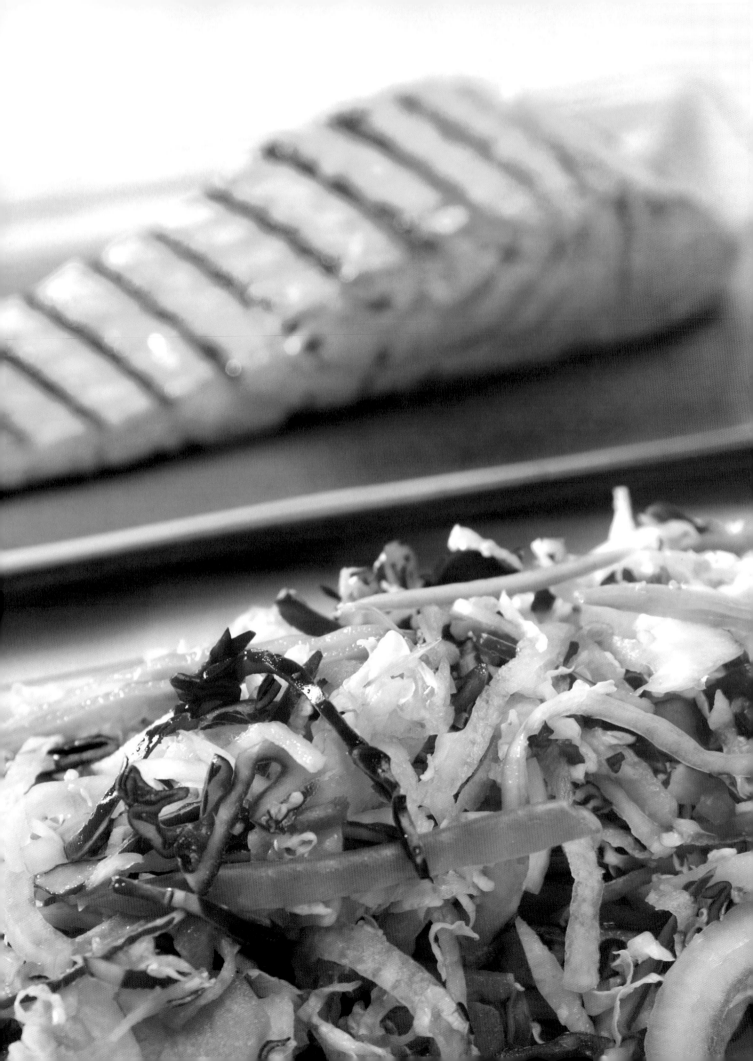

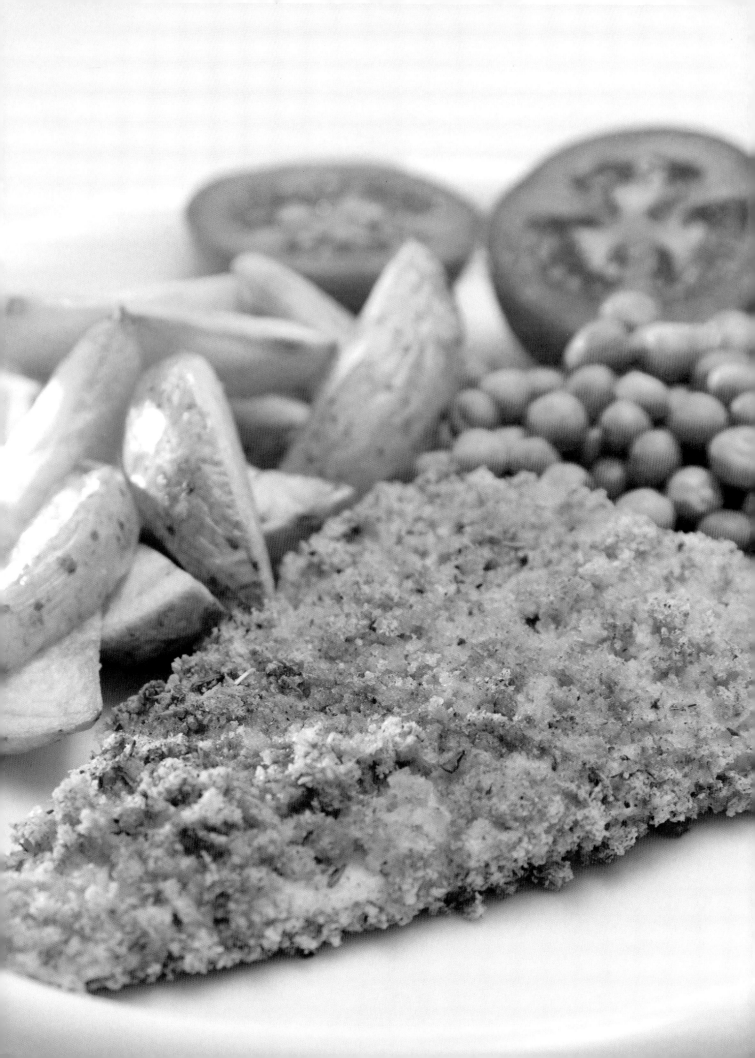

Crispy Oven Fried Cod

Family Favourite

This is served with home-made oven chips for a fish and chip supper that has far less fat than a take-away. To make oven chips, cut potatoes into chunky chips, toss in a little oil and bake for about 40 minutes. Or why not try the chilli oven wedges in the snack section? Don't forget a serving of green vegetables to make the meal nutritionally complete.

Ingredients for 2

50g/2oz day-old bread
without crusts, cut into
cubes
2 cod fillets, skinned
1 tsp olive oil
salt and freshly ground
black pepper
50ml/2fl oz low-fat natural
yoghurt
1 tsp dried mixed herbs
½ tsp paprika

Ingredients for 4

100g/4oz day-old bread
without crusts, cut into
cubes
4 cod fillets, skinned
2 tsp olive oil
salt and freshly ground
black pepper
100ml/3½fl oz low-fat natural
yoghurt
2 tsp dried mixed herbs
1 tsp paprika

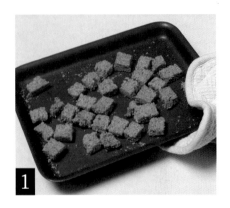

1 Preheat the oven to 180°C/350°F/gas mark 4. Spread the bread cubes on a baking sheet and toast in the oven for 10 minutes. Process to form fine crumbs.

2 Brush the fish with oil and season with a little salt and pepper. Pour the yoghurt into a shallow dish. Add the fish and turn to coat in the yoghurt mixture.

3 Place the crumbs on a plate and stir in the herbs and paprika. Coat the fish in the breadcrumbs.

4 Place the fish in a single layer on a lightly greased baking sheet.

5 Bake for 30 minutes or until the fish is cooked through.

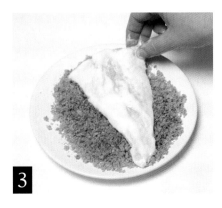

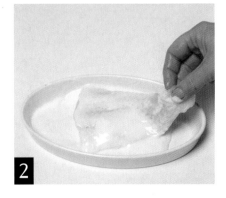

Grilled Plaice with Spinach Rice

This is a complete meal in one.

Ingredients for 2

2 plaice fillets

Spinach rice:

1 tsp olive oil
1 small onion, chopped
75g/3oz brown rice
225ml/8fl oz vegetable stock
**125g/4½oz frozen chopped
  spinach, thawed and
  drained**
2 tsp pine nuts, toasted
**salt and freshly ground
  black pepper**

Ingredients for 4

4 plaice fillets

Spinach rice:

2 tsp olive oil
1 onion, chopped
175g/6oz brown rice
450ml/¾pt vegetable stock
**250g/9oz frozen chopped
  spinach, thawed and
  drained**
1 tbsp pine nuts, toasted
**salt and freshly ground
  black pepper**

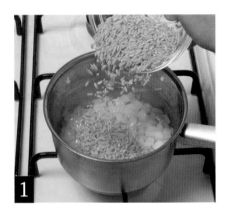

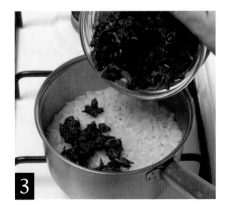

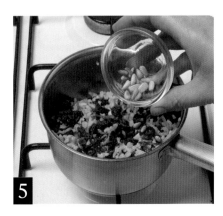

1 To make the rice, heat the oil in a saucepan and sauté the onion for 5 minutes until beginning to brown. Stir in the rice and cook for 1 minute.

2 Add the stock and bring to the boil. Stir, cover and simmer for 30 minutes until almost cooked.

3 Add the spinach to the pan, cover and continue to cook while cooking the fish.

4 Place the fish under a preheated grill, skin-side up, and cook for 2 minutes. Turn over and cook for a further 2–3 minutes until the flesh flakes easily.

5 Stir the pine nuts into the rice and spoon the rice on to a serving plate. Serve with the fish.

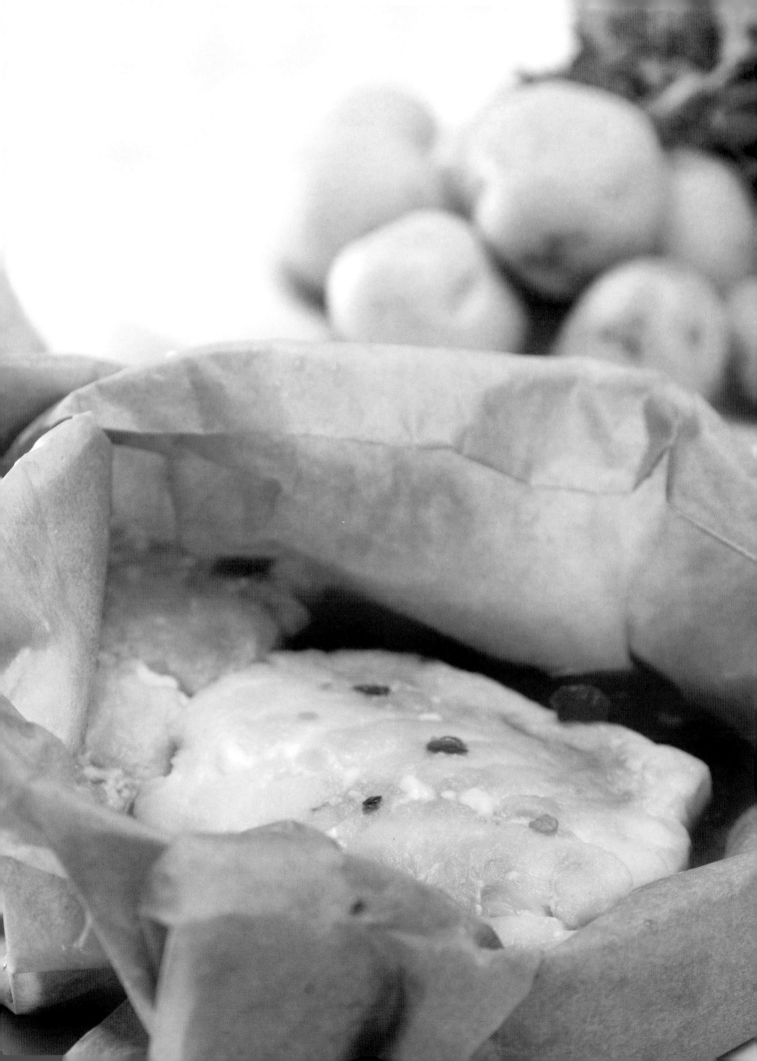

Fish with Chilli & Soy

Hot and spicy

This just has to be the simplest fish dish I know, and yet it is extremely tasty. You can use any fish, fillet or on the bone. Why not try sea bass, cod, trout, tuna, salmon or red mullet?

Ingredients for 2

2 portions of fish of your choice
2 tbsp soy sauce
2 tbsp sweet chilli sauce

Ingredients for 4

4 portions of fish of your choice
4 tbsp soy sauce
4 tbsp sweet chilli sauce

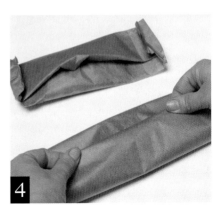

1 Place each fish portion on a double sheet of greaseproof paper or baking parchment.

2 Combine the soy and sweet chilli sauce.

3 Pour a little of the soy and chilli mixture over each fish.

4 Wrap up parcels to enclose the fish and steam for 10–20 minutes depending on the thickness of the fish. The fish will flake easily when cooked.

5 Serve with a salad and new potatoes or crusty bread.

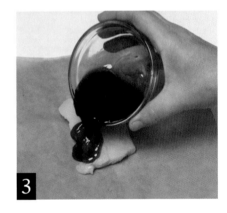

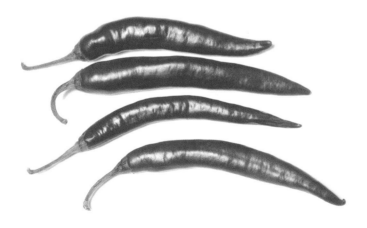

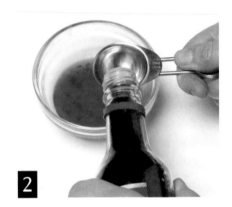

Tandoori Chicken

Hot and spicy

Serve with brown rice and a tomato and onion salad for a well-balanced meal.

Ingredients for 2

2 chicken breasts, skinned
  and boned
100g/4oz low-fat natural
  yoghurt
1 tsp paprika
1 tsp chilli powder
½ tsp ground coriander
½ tsp ground cumin
½ tsp mustard powder
¼ tsp ground ginger
¼ tsp ground turmeric
coriander to garnish,
  optional

Ingredients for 4

4 chicken breasts, skinned
  and boned
225g/8oz low-fat natural
  yoghurt
2 tsp paprika
2 tsp chilli powder
1 tsp ground coriander
1 tsp ground cumin
1 tsp mustard powder
½ tsp ground ginger
½ tsp ground turmeric
coriander to garnish,
  optional

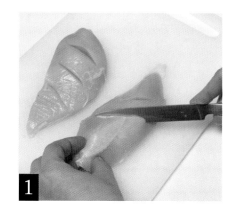

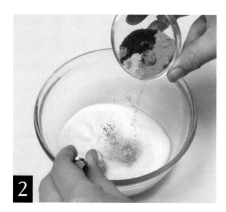

1 Cut two or three slashes into each chicken breast.

2 Place the yoghurt in a bowl and stir in all the spices.

3 Place the chicken in a shallow dish and pour over the yoghurt mixture. Turn until well coated.

4 Allow to marinate for at least 3 hours or overnight if possible.

5 Preheat the oven to 200°C/400°F/gas mark 6.

6 Place the chicken on a trivet over a roasting dish.

7 Bake for 30–35 minutes or until the juices run clear. Garnish with coriander if desired.

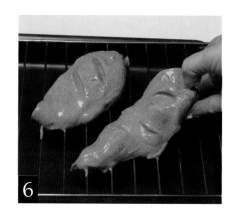

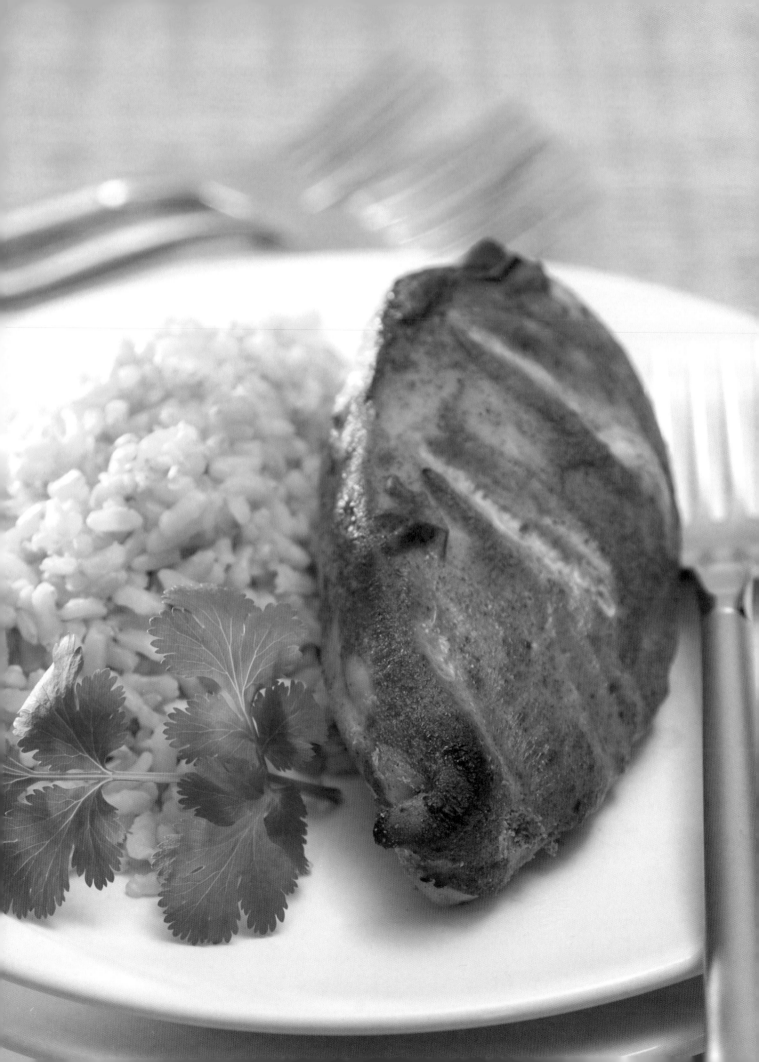

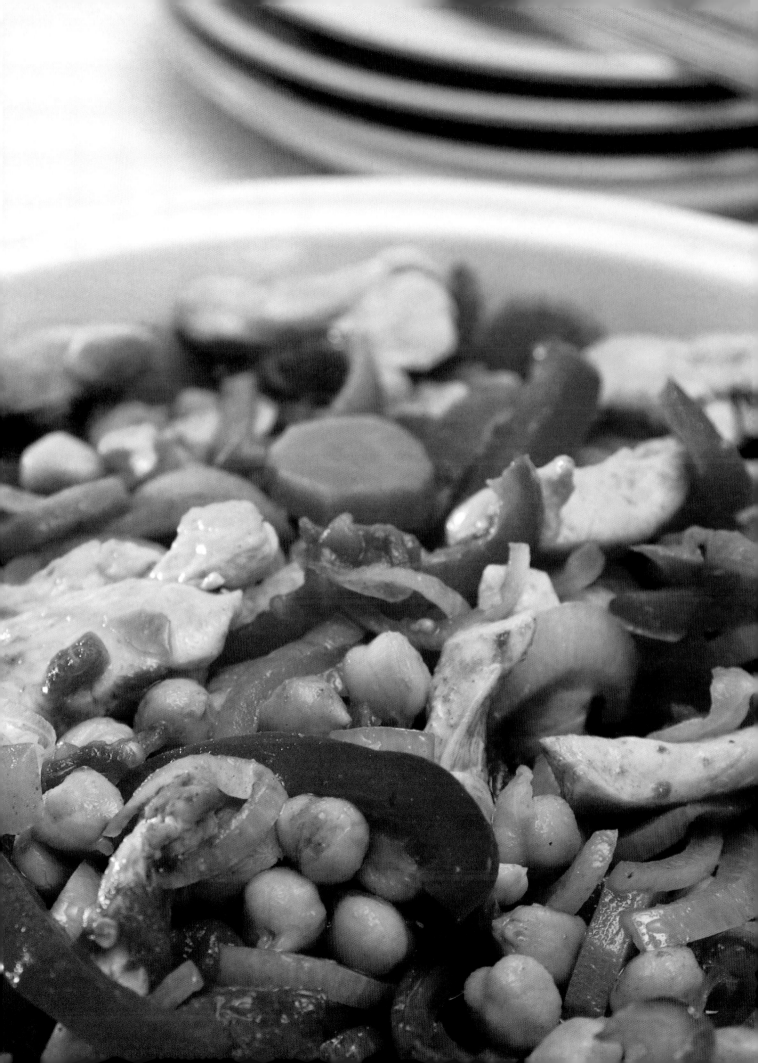

Chicken & Chickpea Casserole

This is a filling casserole. Serve with fresh green vegetables and crusty wholemeal bread.

Ingredients for 2

- 1 large or 2 small chicken breasts, skinned and boned
- 2 tsp olive oil
- 1 small onion, sliced
- 1 clove garlic, chopped
- 1 medium carrot, thinly sliced
- ½ red pepper, seeded and sliced
- ½ green pepper, seeded and sliced
- 2 tsp paprika
- 200g/7oz can chopped tomatoes with herbs
- 75ml/2½fl oz chicken stock
- 200g/7oz can chick peas

Ingredients for 4

- 3 chicken breasts, skinned and boned
- 1 tbsp olive oil
- 1 large onion, sliced
- 2 cloves garlic, chopped
- 2 medium carrots, thinly sliced
- 1 red pepper, seeded and sliced
- 1 green pepper, seeded and sliced
- 2 tsp paprika
- 400g/14oz can chopped tomatoes with herbs
- 150ml/¼pt chicken stock
- 400g/14oz can chick peas

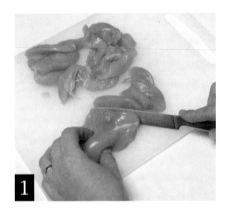

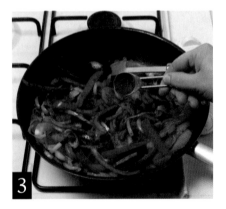

1 Preheat the oven to 180°C/350°F/gas mark 4. Cut the chicken into strips.

2 Heat the oil in a non-stick frying pan and brown the chicken on all sides. Transfer to an ovenproof casserole.

3 Add the onions, garlic, carrot and peppers to the non-stick frying pan and sauté for 5 minutes until softened. Sprinkle over the paprika and cook for 1 minute.

4 Pour in the tomatoes and stock and bring to the boil. Pour over the chicken.

5 Stir in the chick peas.

6 Cover and cook in the centre of the oven for 45 minutes.

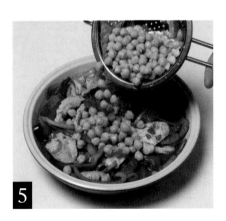

Pepper Crusted Chicken with Salad in an Oriental Dressing

Easy Entertaining

Serve with boiled noodles or new potatoes. If you do not have Szechwan peppercorns you could use black or green peppercorns instead.

Ingredients for 2

2 chicken breasts, skinned and boned
sesame oil
2 tbsp Szechwan peppercorns
50g/2oz herb leaf salad
2 tbsp soy sauce
½ tsp dark muscovado sugar
1 tsp lime juice

Ingredients for 4

4 chicken breasts, skinned and boned
sesame oil
3 tbsp Szechwan peppercorns
100g/4oz herb leaf salad
4 tbsp soy sauce
1 tsp dark muscovado sugar
1 tbsp lime juice

1 Place the chicken between two sheets of cling wrap and flatten with a meat mallet or rolling pin.

2 Brush the top of the chicken with a little sesame oil.

3 Crush the peppercorns and press on the top of the chicken.

4 Heat a heavy based non-stick frying pan griddle or barbecue and cook for 3-4 minutes each side, or until cooked through.

5 Meanwhile, place the salad leaves in a serving dish.

6 Combine the remaining ingredients with 2 (4) tsp sesame oil. Pour over the leaves and toss to coat.

7 Slice the chicken into strips and serve on top of the salad.

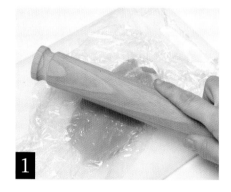

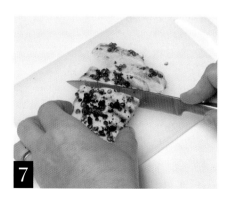

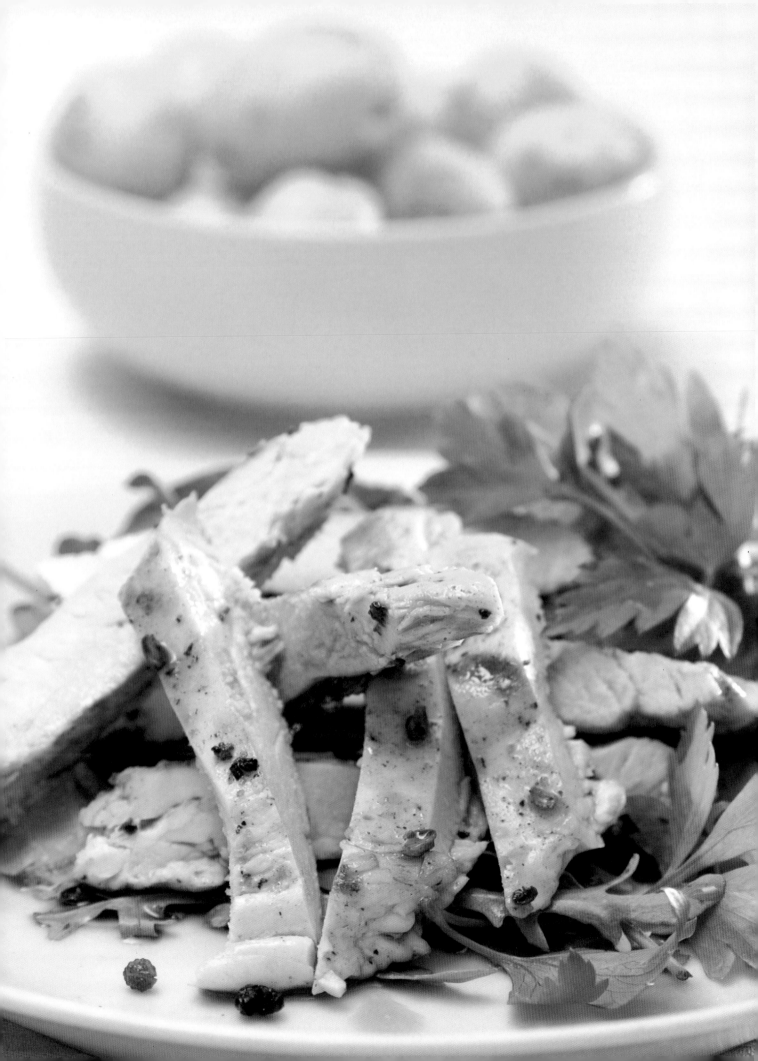

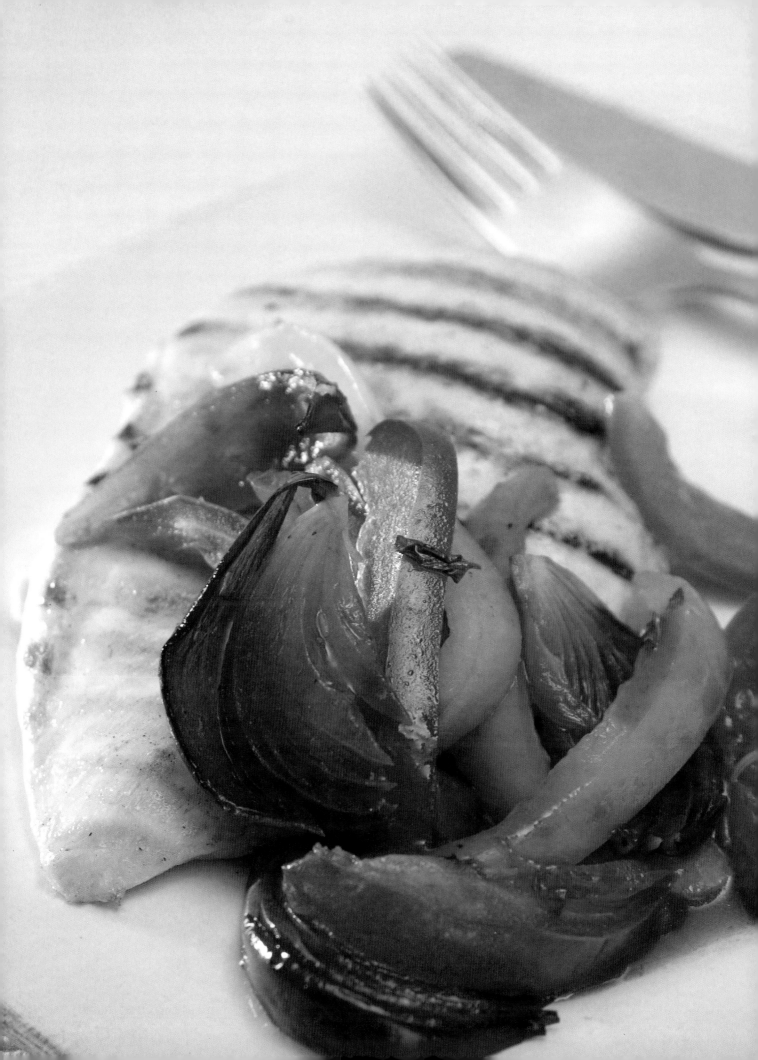

Grilled Chicken with Chunky Pepperonata

Flattening the chicken allows you to cook it more quickly. The cooking time will depend on how thin the chicken is. Griddle pans are great for cooking meat with very little oil – just wipe a little oil on to the surface with kitchen paper before heating. Alternatively grill or use a non-stick frying pan.

Ingredients for 2

2 chicken breasts, skinned
    and boned
salt and freshly ground
    black pepper
1 tsp olive oil
1 small red onion, peeled
    and cut into wedges
1 clove garlic, chopped
½ red pepper, seeded and
    sliced
½ yellow pepper, seeded and
    sliced
1 tomato, seeded and sliced
1-2 tsp fresh oregano or
    marjoram, chopped
75ml/2½fl oz chicken stock
1 tsp tomato purée
potatoes, pasta or bread
    to serve

Ingredients for 4

4 chicken breasts, skinned
    and boned
salt and freshly ground
    black pepper
2 tsp olive oil
1 red onion, peeled and cut
    into wedges
2 cloves garlic, chopped
1 red pepper, seeded and
    sliced
1 yellow pepper, seeded and
    sliced
2 tomatoes, seeded and
    sliced
1 tbsp fresh oregano or
    marjoram, chopped
150ml/¼pt chicken stock
2 tsp tomato purée
potatoes, pasta or bread
    to serve

1 Place the chicken between two sheets of cling wrap and flatten with a meat mallet or rolling pin. Season with salt and pepper and set aside.

2 Heat the oil in a non-stick frying pan and fry the onion for 5 minutes until softened, then stir in the garlic.

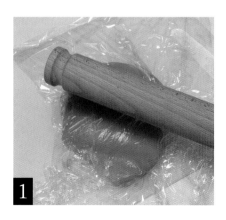

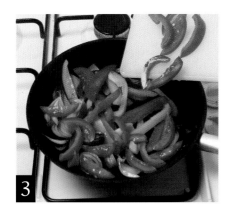

3 Add the peppers and cook for 3 minutes. Stir in the tomatoes, herbs, stock and purée.

4 Bring to the boil. Reduce the heat and simmer gently for 15 minutes.

5 Meanwhile heat a griddle pan, and cook the chicken under the hot grill for 3–4 minutes each side, until the juices run clear. You may need to do this in two batches.

6 Serve the chicken with the pepperonata, pasta, bread or potatoes.

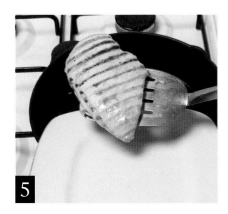

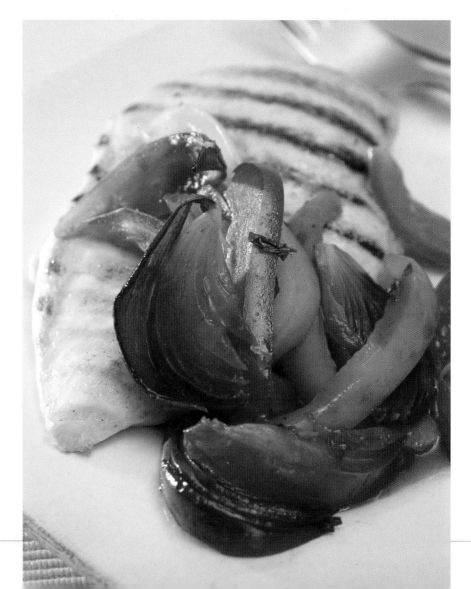

Marinated Lamb with Lemon Couscous

Don't skimp on the herbs as they add lots of flavour to the couscous. Garnish with coriander.

Ingredients for 2

2 lamb rump steaks
salt and freshly ground
  black pepper

Marinade:

grated juice and zest ¼
  lemon
1 tsp olive oil
½ red chilli, seeded and
  chopped
2 tsp fresh coriander,
  chopped

Lemon couscous:

75g/3oz couscous
grated juice and zest ½ lemon
2 tsp olive oil
3 tbsp fresh coriander,
  chopped

Ingredients for 4

4 lamb rump steaks
salt and freshly ground
  black pepper

Marinade:

grated juice and zest ½
  lemon
2 tsp olive oil
1 red chilli, seeded and
  chopped
4 tsp fresh coriander,
  chopped

Lemon couscous:

175g/6oz couscous
grated juice and zest 1 lemon
4 tsp olive oil
6 tbsp fresh coriander,
  chopped

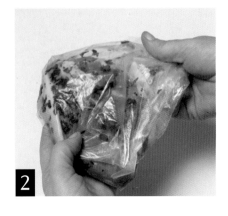

2

1 Season the lamb with salt and pepper.

2 Place the lemon juice and zest, olive oil, chilli and coriander in a strong polythene bag and shake to combine. Add the lamb. Seal and shake until well coated.

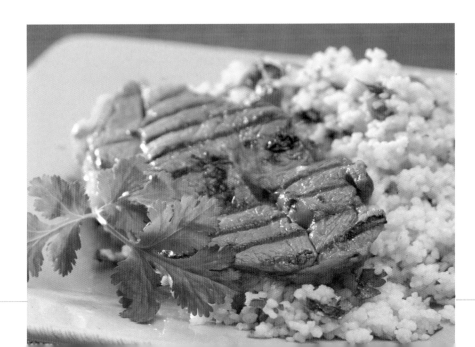

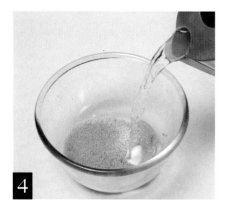

3 Allow to marinate for at least 1 hour or up to 24 hours in the refrigerator.

4 To make the couscous, place in a bowl and cover with 1cm/½in of cold water. Allow to stand for 30 minutes. Drain well and mix with the remaining couscous ingredients. Season well.

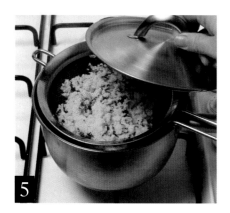

5 Place the soaked couscous in a sieve over a saucepan of gently simmering water. Cover and steam for 10 minutes.

6 Meanwhile, remove the lamb from the marinade. Cook under a hot grill or on a ridged griddle pan for 4–6 minutes each side, depending on how well cooked you like your lamb.

7 Serve with the lemon couscous.

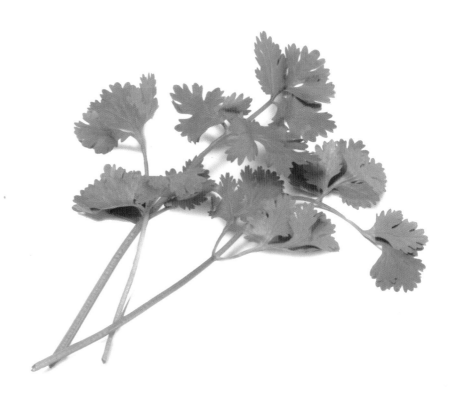

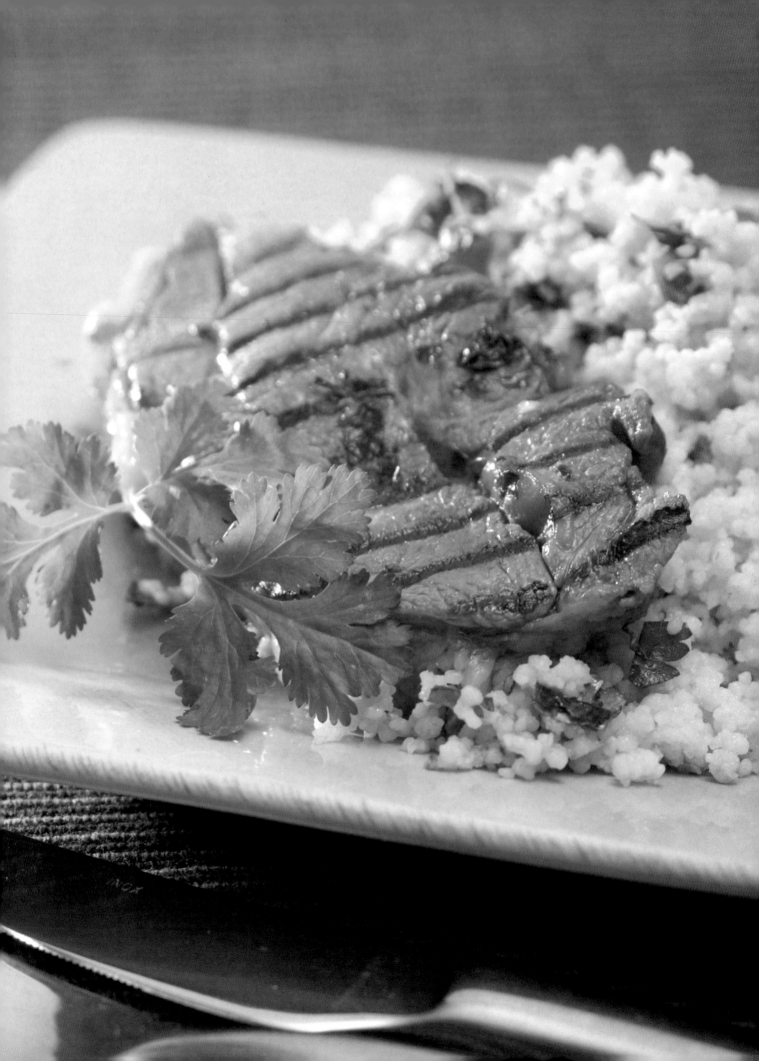

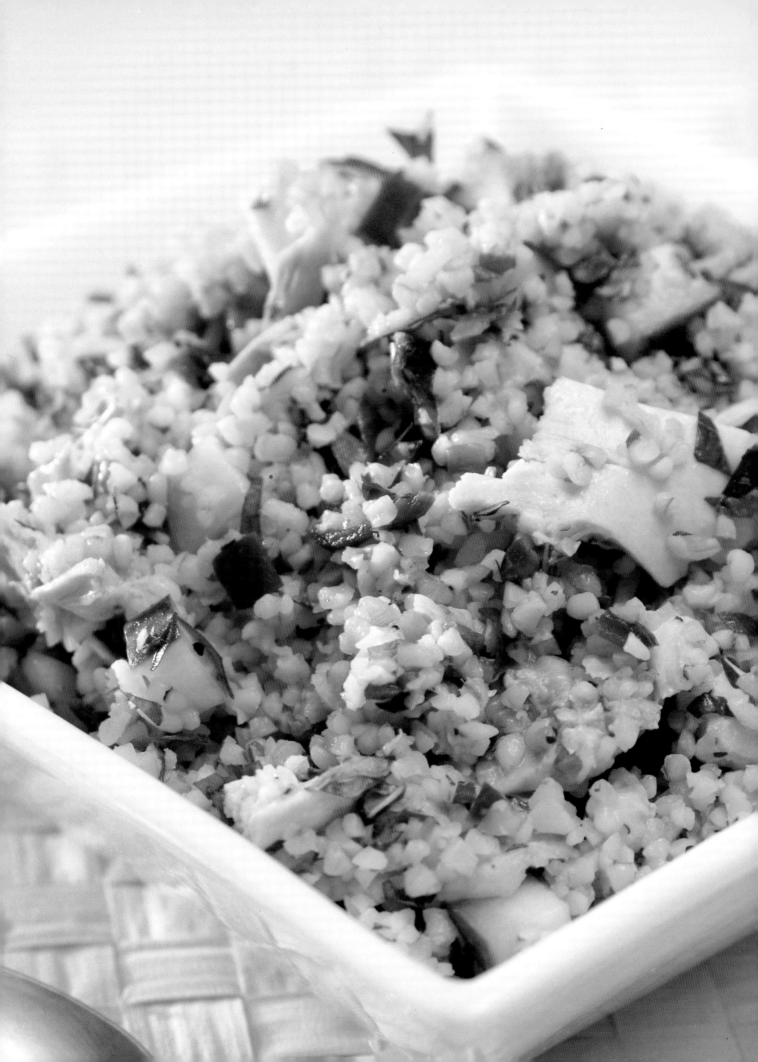

Chicken with Tabouleh

Packed with lots of fresh herbs, this summer dish is full of flavour. You can add chopped peppers for extra colour and flavour, or keep it simple. Don't forget to remove the skin from the chicken thighs to reduce the fat content.

Ingredients for 2

3 cooked chicken thighs
300ml/½pt vegetable stock
100g/4oz bulgur wheat
2 tsp olive oil
1 red onion, finely chopped
2 cloves garlic, chopped
grated zest and juice 1
  lemon
50g/2oz cucumber, seeded
  and chopped
2 tbsp flat leaf parsley,
  chopped
2 tbsp fresh mint, chopped

Ingredients for 4

6 cooked chicken thighs
600ml/1pt vegetable stock
225g/8oz bulgur wheat
2 tsp olive oil
1 red onion, finely chopped
2 cloves garlic, chopped
grated zest and juice 1
  lemon
100g/4oz cucumber, seeded
  and chopped
4 tbsp flat leaf parsley,
  chopped
4 tbsp fresh mint, chopped

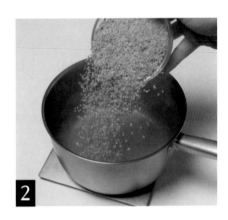

1 Skin and bone the chicken. Cut into bite-size pieces.

2 Bring the stock to the boil. Remove from the heat and stir in the bulgur wheat. Cover and allow to stand for at least 20 minutes.

3 Meanwhile heat the oil in a non-stick frying pan and fry the onion and garlic over a medium heat for 5–10 minutes until tender. Allow to cool.

4 Stir in the lemon zest and juice and season well.

5 Fluff up the bulgur wheat with a fork. Add the chicken, cucumber and herbs.

6 Pour over the onion mixture and toss together until well combined.

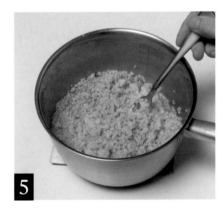

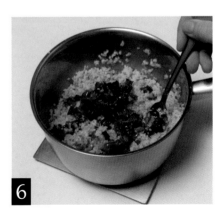

Oven Baked Pork with Roasted Chilli Tomato Salsa

Hot and spicy

I find pork can be a little dry, so I like to serve it with a sauce or salsa. This spicy salsa is perfect. Serve with new potatoes and fresh green beans for a well-balanced meal. Use regular paprika if you cannot get smoked paprika.

Ingredients for 2

2 lean pork chops
salt and freshly ground
   black pepper
2 plum tomatoes
½ small red onion, chopped
1 red chilli, seeded and
   chopped
2 tsp olive oil
1 tsp lime juice
¼ tsp smoked paprika
potatoes, pasta or rice to
   serve

Ingredients for 4

4 lean pork chops
salt and freshly ground
   black pepper
4 plum tomatoes
1 small red onion, chopped
1 or 2 red chilli, seeded and
   chopped
1 tbsp olive oil
2 tsp lime juice
½ tsp smoked paprika
potatoes, pasta or rice to
   serve

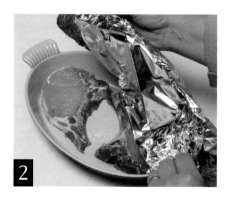

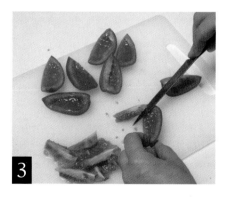

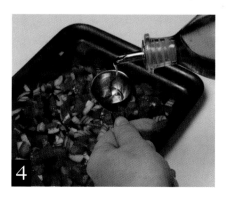

1 Preheat the oven to 180°C/350°F/gas mark 4.

2 Place the pork in a lightly oiled, shallow baking dish. Season with salt and pepper and cover the dish with foil. Bake in the oven for 35 minutes or until the juices run clear.

3 Meanwhile cut the tomatoes in half, scoop out the seeds and discard. Dice the flesh. Place on a small baking sheet with the onion and chilli.

4 Drizzle with olive oil and roast for 15 minutes.

5 Transfer the roasted tomatoes, onion and chilli to a bowl and stir in the lime juice and paprika. Chill until required.

6 Serve the pork with potatoes, pasta or rice, with the salsa on the side.

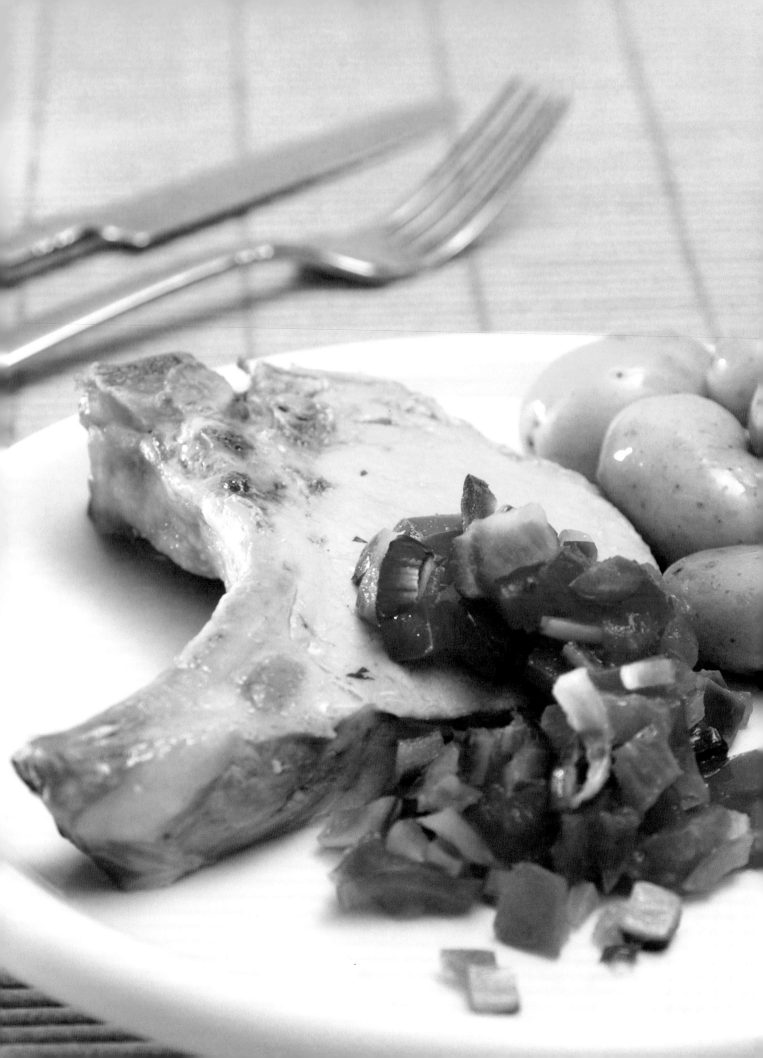

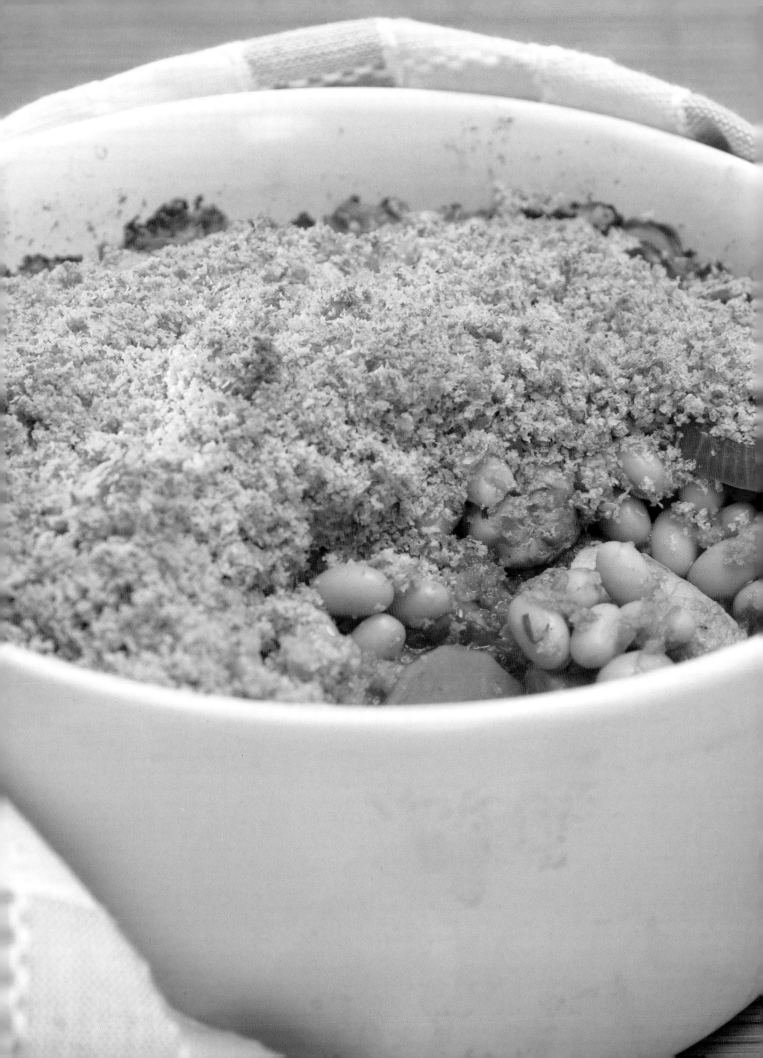

Pork Cassoulet

Canned beans are very convenient, but if you use beans a lot you will find it more economical to buy dried beans. These can be soaked and cooked in advance and frozen in usable portions.

Ingredients for 2

1 tsp olive oil
250g/9oz pork fillet, sliced
1 onion, sliced
1 carrot, sliced
1 clove garlic, chopped
75ml2½fl oz red wine
200g/7oz can chopped
    tomatoes
1 bay leaf
½ tsp dried thyme
½ tsp dried rosemary
2 cloves
salt and freshly ground
    black pepper
400g/14oz can haricot beans,
    rinsed and drained
40g/1½oz fresh wholemeal
    bread crumbs

Ingredients for 4

2 tsp olive oil
500g/1lb 2oz pork fillet,
    sliced
2 onions sliced
2 carrots, sliced
2 cloves garlic, chopped
150ml/¼pt red wine
400g/14oz can chopped
    tomatoes
2 bay leaf
1 tsp dried thyme
1 tsp dried rosemary
4 cloves
salt and freshly ground
    black pepper
2 x 400g/14oz cans haricot
    beans, rinsed and drained
75g/3oz fresh wholemeal
    bread crumbs

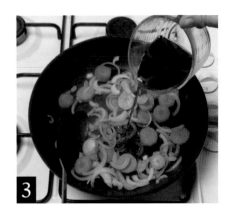

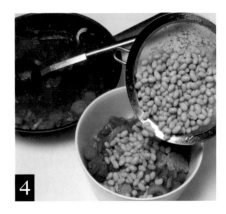

1 Preheat the oven to 180°C/350°F/gas mark 4. Heat the oil in a non-stick frying pan and fry the meat until browned on both sides. Remove from the pan.

2 Add the onion and carrot and sauté for 4–5 minutes until just softened. Add the garlic and sauté for 1 minute.

3 Add the wine, bring to the boil and simmer for 1–2 minutes. Then add the tomatoes, herbs and cloves and return to the boil. Season with salt and pepper.

4 Layer the pork, vegetable mixture and beans in a deep ovenproof casserole.

5 Sprinkle the breadcrumbs on top and bake for 50–60 minutes.

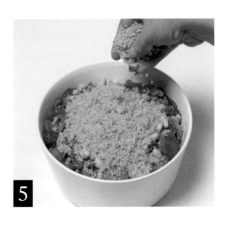

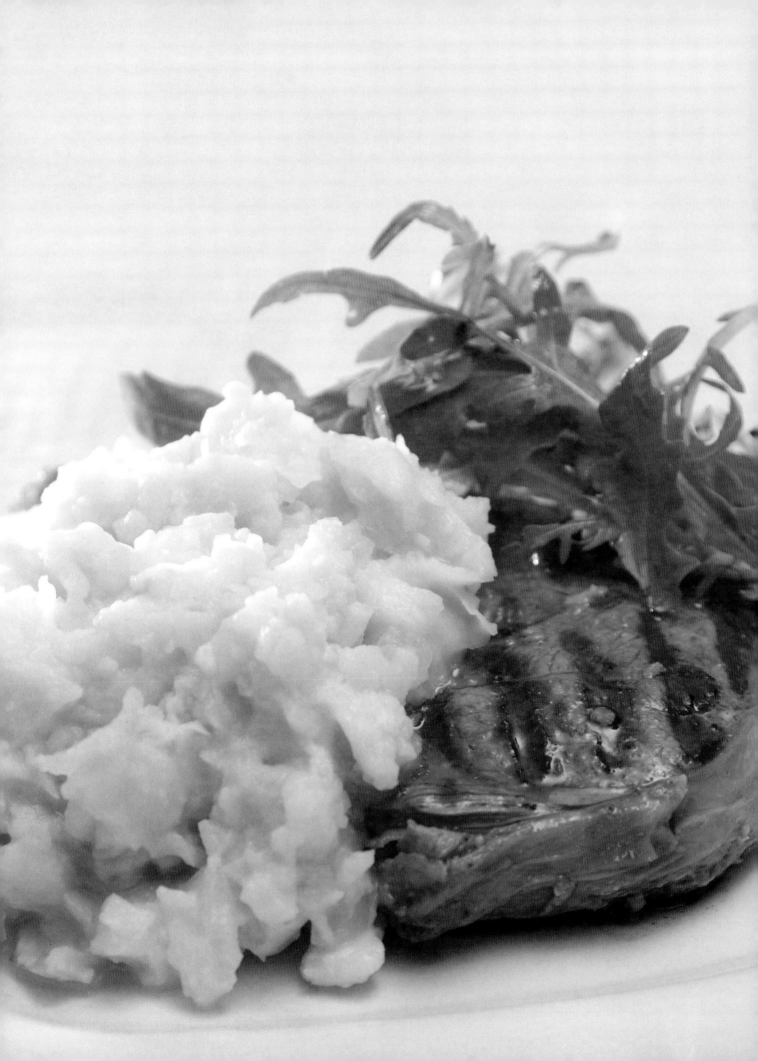

Marinated Lamb with White Bean Mash

Easy Entertaining

Try this great alternative to potato mash. Beans have loads of soluble flavour so the energy is released slowly, perfect for people with diabetes.

Ingredients for 2

2 lamb leg steaks
½ tsp olive oil
1 tbsp lemon juice
1 clove garlic, crushed
1 tsp chopped fresh thyme

Bean mash:

1 tsp olive oil
1 small onion, chopped
1 clove garlic, crushed
1 tsp fresh thyme, chopped
75 ml/2½fl oz skimmed or
    semi-skimmed milk
400g/14oz can haricot beans,
    rinsed and drained

Ingredients for 4

4 lamb leg steaks
1 tsp olive oil
2 tbsp lemon juice
2 cloves garlic, crushed
2 tsp chopped fresh thyme

Bean mash:

2 tsp olive oil
1 onion, chopped
2 cloves garlic, crushed
2 tsp fresh thyme, chopped
150ml/¼pt skimmed or
    semi-skimmed milk
2 x 400g/14oz cans haricot
    beans, rinsed and drained

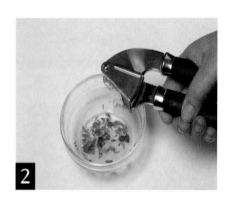

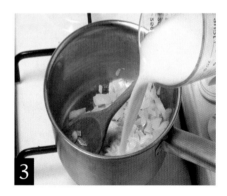

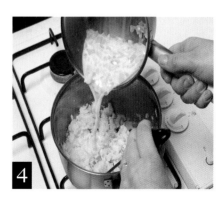

1 Place the lamb steak in a shallow non-metallic dish.

2 Mix together the oil, lemon juice, garlic and thyme and pour over the meat. Allow to marinate for at least 1 hour or for up to 24 hours.

3 To make the mash, heat the oil in a saucepan and gently sauté the onion for 5 minutes until soft. Add the garlic and cook for 1 minute.

Add the milk, and heat until piping hot.

4 Meanwhile cook the beans in boiling water for 5 minutes until piping hot, drain and mash. Beat in the onion mixture and keep warm.

5 Remove the lamb from the marinade. Cook under a preheated grill or on a ridged griddle pan for 4–6 minutes a side. Serve with the bean mash.

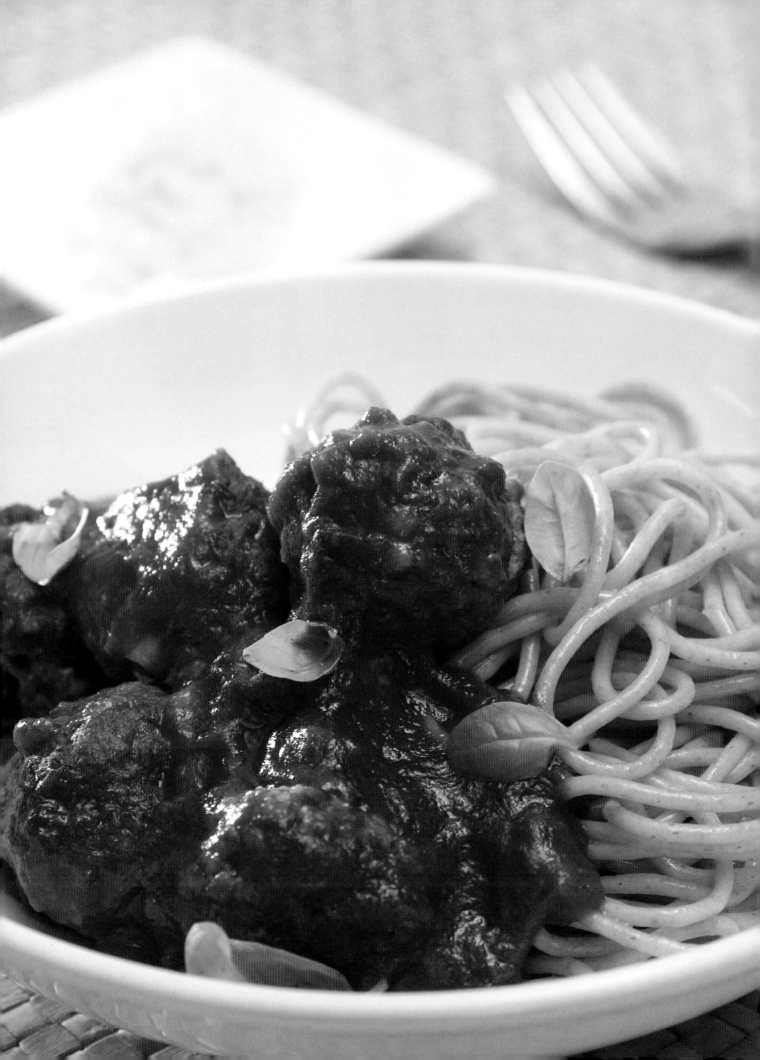

Meatballs with Spaghetti

Family Favourite

This is a classic Italian dish – given the healthy treatment. Sprinkle a little Parmesan cheese and some fresh basil leaves over the top. Serve a mixed salad with or after the pasta to make a nutritionally complete meal.

Ingredients for 2

- 250g/9oz extra-lean mince beef
- fresh wholemeal breadcrumbs
- shallot, finely chopped
- clove garlic, chopped
- ½ tsp dried oregano
- 2 tsp Parmesan cheese, grated
- 1 egg yolk
- salt and freshly ground black pepper
- 1 tsp olive oil
- 250g/9oz passata
- 200g/7oz wholemeal spaghetti

Ingredients for 4

- 500g/1lb 2oz extra lean mince beef
- fresh wholemeal breadcrumbs
- shallots, finely chopped
- cloves garlic, chopped
- 1 tsp dried oregano
- 1 tbsp Parmesan cheese, grated
- 1 egg yolk plus 1 tbsp water
- salt and freshly ground black pepper
- 2 tsp olive oil
- 500g/1lb 2oz jar passata
- 400g/14oz wholemeal spaghetti

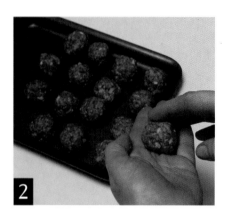

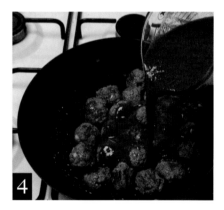

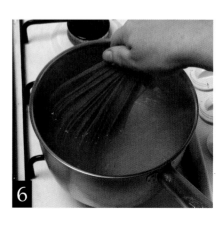

1 Place the beef, breadcrumbs, onion, shallot, garlic, oregano, cheese and egg yolk (and water) in a mixing bowl. Season with salt and pepper and mix until well blended.

2 Form into small balls.

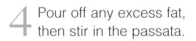

3 Heat the oil in a large, non-stick frying pan and fry the balls until browned on all sides.

4 Pour off any excess fat, then stir in the passata.

5 Bring to the boil, reduce the heat and simmer, covered, for 20 minutes.

6 Cook the spaghetti in plenty of lightly salted boiling water for 12 minutes, or as directed on the packet. Drain and serve with the meatballs

Pot Roast Beef

Family Favourite

Slow cooking the beef makes it very tender, but remember to spoon off any fat that forms on top of the gravy. I like to serve this with plenty of vegetables and potatoes. Mashed potatoes are great to soak up the gravy.

Ingredients for 3-4

700g/1½lb topside of beef
salt and freshly ground black
   pepper
2 tsp sunflower oil
2 onions, sliced
½ tsp light muscovado sugar
150ml/¼pt red wine
150ml/¼pt beef stock
1 bay leaf
1 sprig fresh thyme

Ingredients for 6-8

1.3kg/3lb topside of beef
salt and freshly ground black
   pepper
4 tsp sunflower oil
3 large onions, sliced
1 tsp light muscovado sugar
300ml/½pt red wine
300ml/½pt beef stock
2 bay leaves
2 sprigs fresh thyme

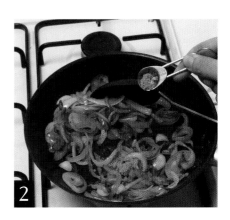

1 Preheat the oven to 170°C/325°F/gas mark 3. Season meat.

2 Heat half the oil in a large, non-stick frying pan and fry the onions over a low heat for 10 minutes until beginning to turn golden. Stir in the sugar and cook for 1–2 minutes more.

3 Remove from the heat and spread over the base of a large, deep ovenproof casserole. Wipe out the pan with a pad of kitchen paper. Take care not to burn yourself as the pan will be very hot.

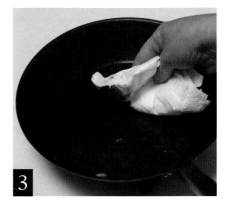

4 Heat the remaining oil in the non-stick frying pan and fry the meat briskly on all sides over a high heat until browned and sealed. Place the meat on top of the onion.

5 Add the wine, stock and herbs. Cover and cook in the centre of the oven for 2½ hours.

6 Remove the meat from the pan and discard the herb sprigs.

7 Carve the meat and serve with the onion gravy spooned over.

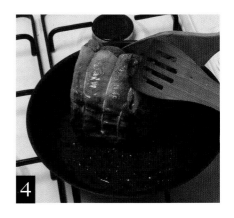

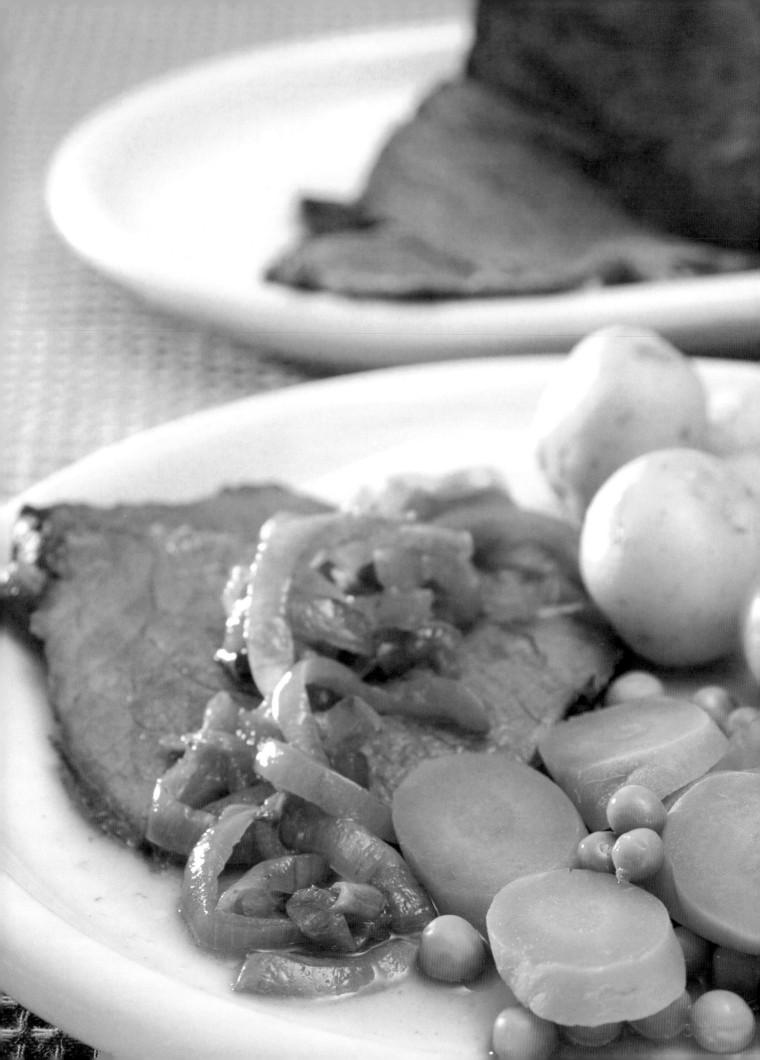

Beef & Noodle Stir Fry

Quick and Easy

Stir fries are ideal for people with diabetes, especially when you need to throw a meal together in a short space of time. Despite its title, stir fry uses very little oil – resist if you feel the urge to add extra and use a little stock or water instead.

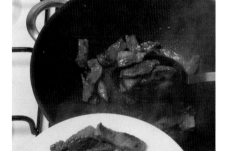

Ingredients for 2

100g/4oz rump steak, cut into thin strips
1 tsp sunflower oil
2 spring onions, sliced diagonally
100g/4oz mangetout
1 carrot, sliced diagonally
25 g/1oz water chestnuts, sliced (optional)
50g/2oz can pineapple chunks in natural juice (drained weight)
1 tsp cornflour mixed with a little water
1 tsp white wine vinegar
2 tsp soy sauce
2 tbsp pineapple juice from the can
200g/7oz fresh egg noodles

Ingredients for 4

225g/8oz rump steak, cut into thin strips
2 tsp sunflower oil
4 spring onions, sliced diagonally
200g/7oz mangetout
2 carrots, sliced diagonally
50g/2oz water chestnuts, sliced (optional)
100g/4oz can pineapple chunks in natural juice (drained weight)
2 tsp cornflour mixed with a little water
2 tsp white wine vinegar
1 tbsp soy sauce
4 tbsp pineapple juice from the can
400g/14oz fresh egg noodles

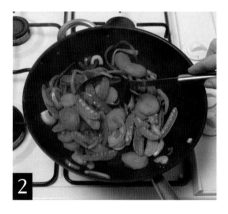

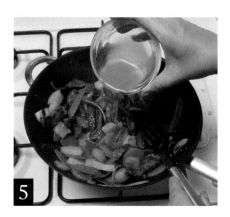

1 Toss the meat with the oil until well coated. Heat a wok, add the meat and stir fry briskly until browned. Remove from the pan.

2 Add the spring onions, mangetout, carrots and water chestnuts, if using, and cook for 3–4 minutes.

3 Return the meat to the wok and add the pineapple. Cook for 1–2 minutes.

4 Mix the cornflour with the vinegar and soy, then stir in the pineapple juice.

5 Add to the wok and cook, stirring until the sauce thickens.

6 Meanwhile cook the noodles in boiling water for 3–4 minutes, drain and add to the wok. Toss together and serve immediately.

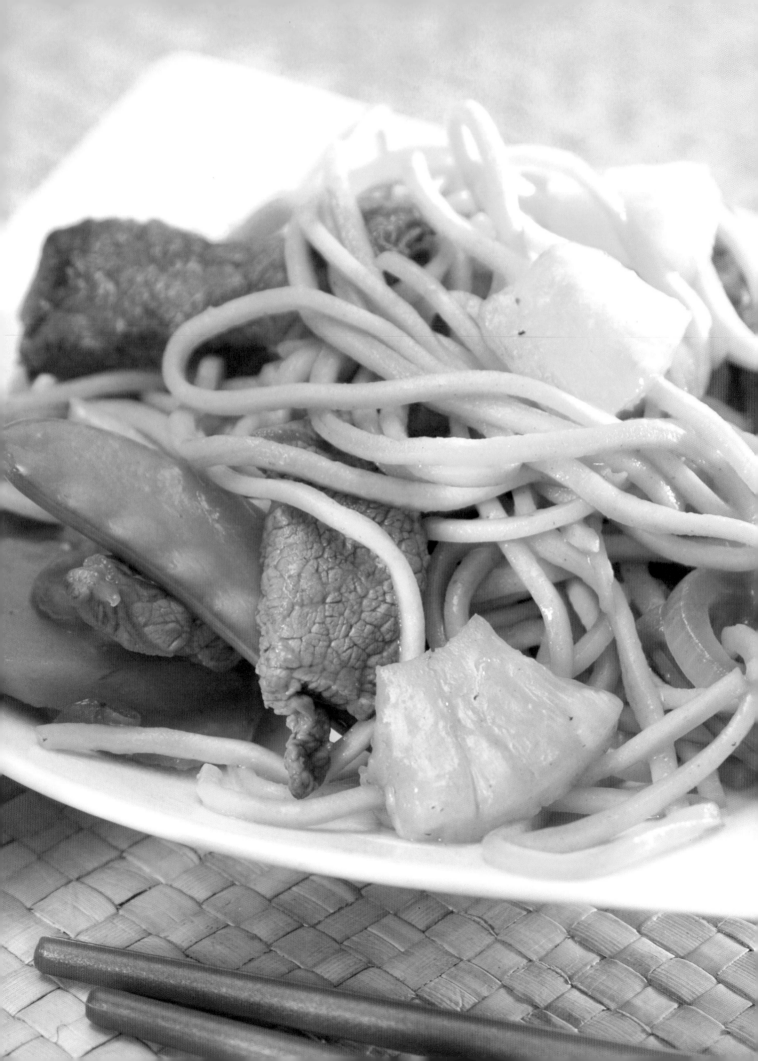

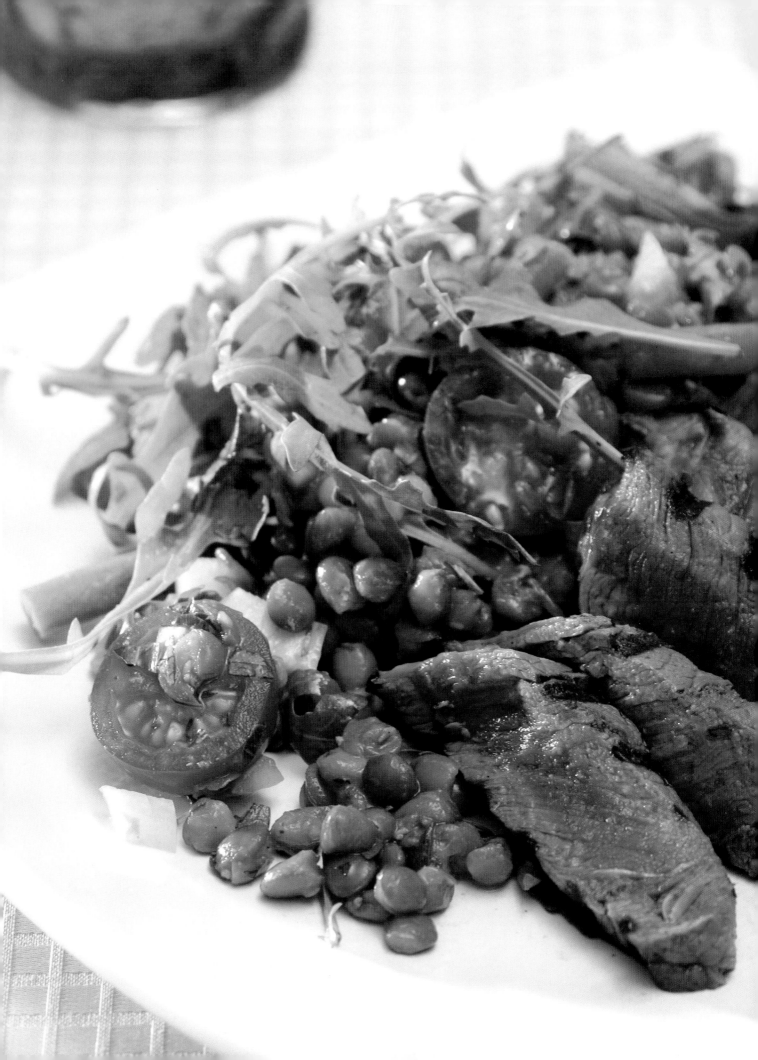

Steak with Lentil & Tomato Salad

While red meat contains saturated fat it is also an important source of iron, so should not be eliminated from the diet completely. However, try to choose very lean pieces. Eaten occasionally with plenty of carbohydrate and fresh vegetables it is a very nutritious meal.

Ingredients for 2

2 x 150-175g fillet, rump or
   sirloin steaks
salt and freshly ground
   black pepper
125g/4½oz fresh green
beans, trimmed
400g/14oz can lentils,
   drained and rinsed
1 shallot, chopped
75g/3oz cherry tomatoes,
   halved
2 tbsp fresh parsley, chopped
small handful basil leaves,
   torn into pieces
2 tbsp low-fat vinaigrette
   dressing
25g/1oz rocket leaves

Ingredients for 4

4 x 150-175g fillet, rump or
   sirloin steaks
salt and freshly ground
   black pepper
250g/9oz fresh green beans,
   trimmed
2 x 400g/14oz can lentils,
   drained and rinsed
2 shallots, chopped
175g/6oz cherry tomatoes,
   halved
4 tbsp fresh parsley, chopped
handful basil leaves, torn
   into pieces
4 tbsp low-fat vinaigrette
   dressing
50g/2oz rocket leaves

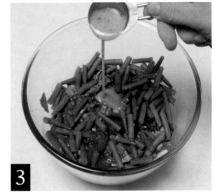

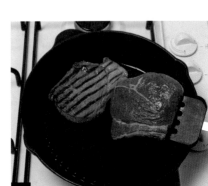

1 Season the steak with salt and pepper.

2 Cut the green beans into short lengths and blanch in boiling water for 2 minutes. Drain and refresh under running cold water.

3 Place the lentils, green beans, shallots, tomatoes and herbs in a large bowl. Sprinkle over the salad dressing and toss until well combined.

4 Heat a griddle pan over a high heat, add the steak and cook for 2–4 minutes each side, depending on how well done you like your steak. Allow to rest for 3 minutes. Alternatively cook under a hot grill.

5 Toss the rocket leaves into the salad and serve with the steak.

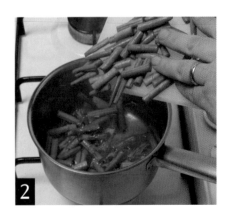

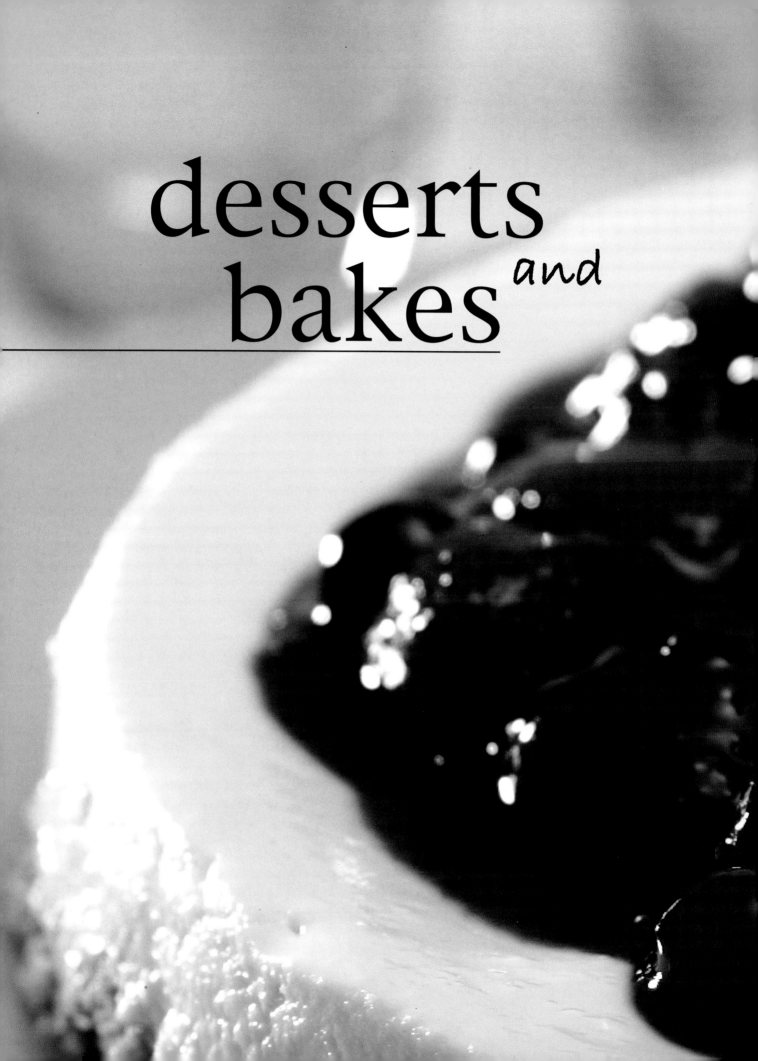

desserts and bakes

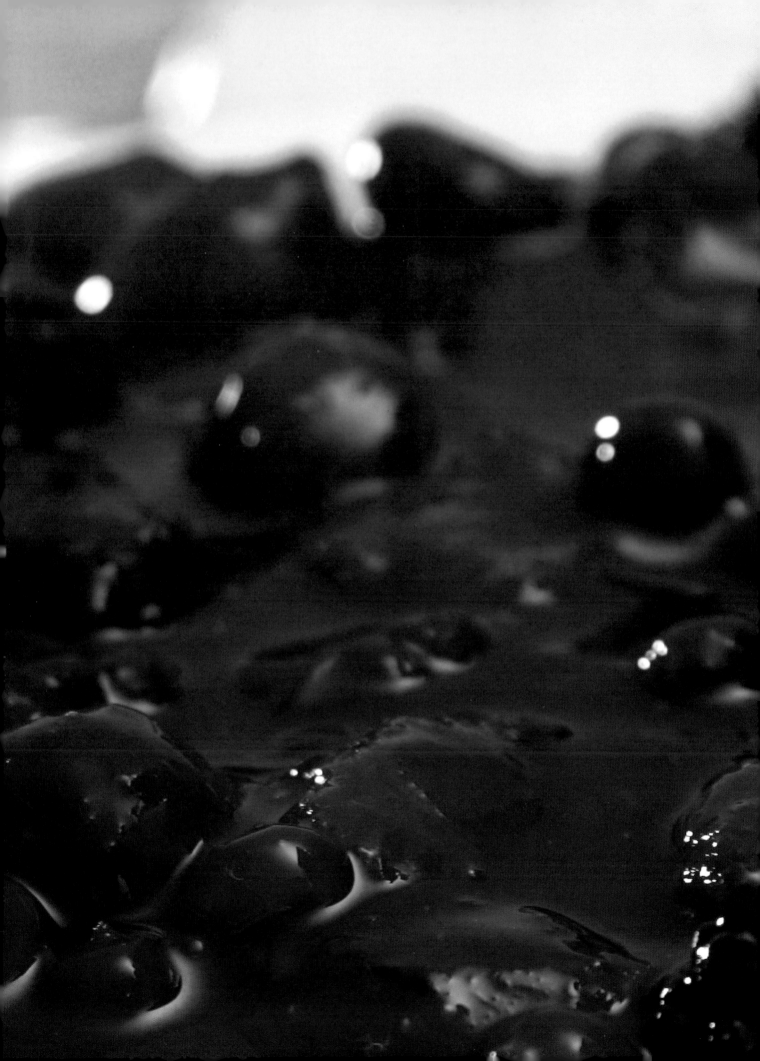

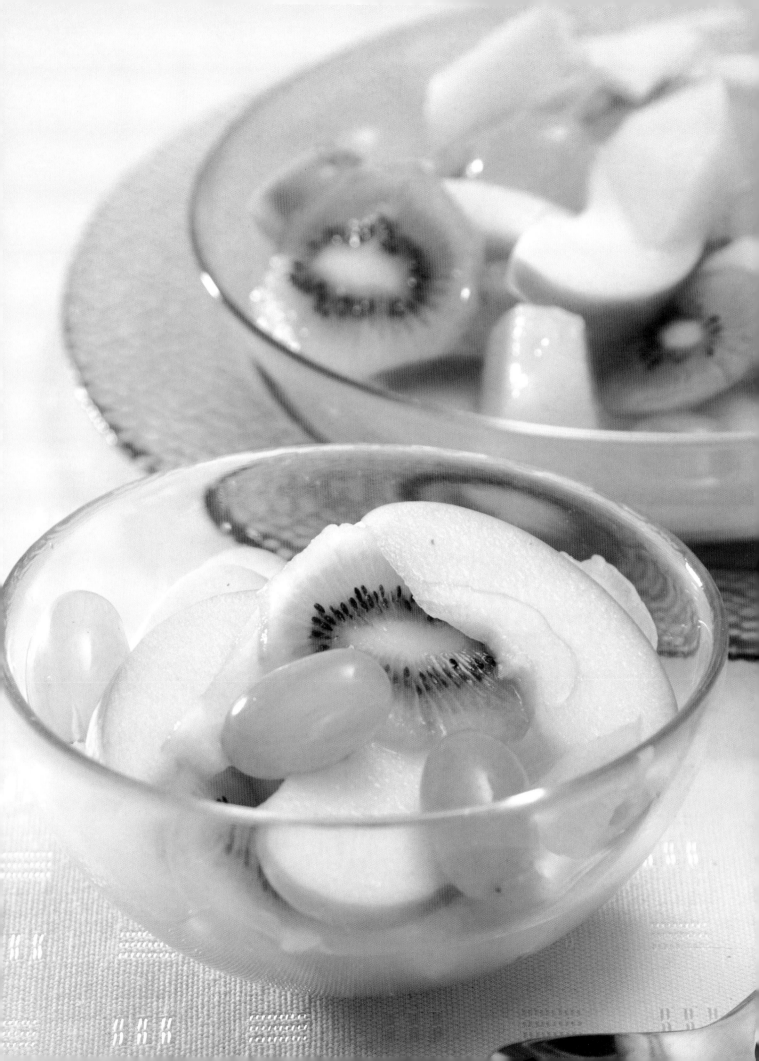

Green Fruit Salad

Easy Entertaining

It is important to eat at least five portions of fruit and vegetables a day for a healthy diet. Fruit salad is therefore a great dessert. Keeping the fruit to one colour tone gives it a more sophisticated appearance, making it ideal when entertaining.

Ingredients for 4-6

½ galia or ¼ honeydew melon
1 kiwi fruit
1 pear
1 green eating apple
50g/2oz green grapes
150ml/¼pt apple juice
2 tbsp orange flavoured
    liqueur (optional)

Ingredients for 6-8

1 galia or ½ honeydew melon
2 kiwi fruits
2 pears
2 green eating apples
100g/4oz green grapes
300ml/½pt apple juice
4 tbsp orange flavoured
    liqueur (optional)

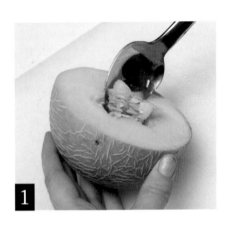

1 Cut the melon in half and scoop out the seeds. Cut into slices and peel, then cut into bite-size chunks.

2 Peel the kiwi and slice crossways. Peel, core and slice the pear.

3 Core and slice the apple. Place all the fruit in a large serving bowl. Pour over the apple juice, add the orange liqueur if using, and toss to combine.

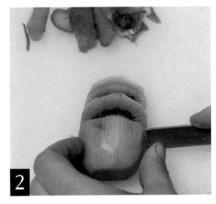

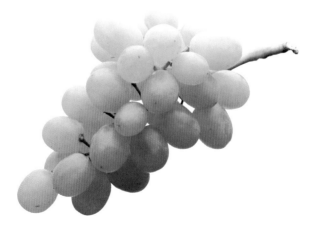

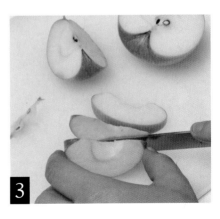

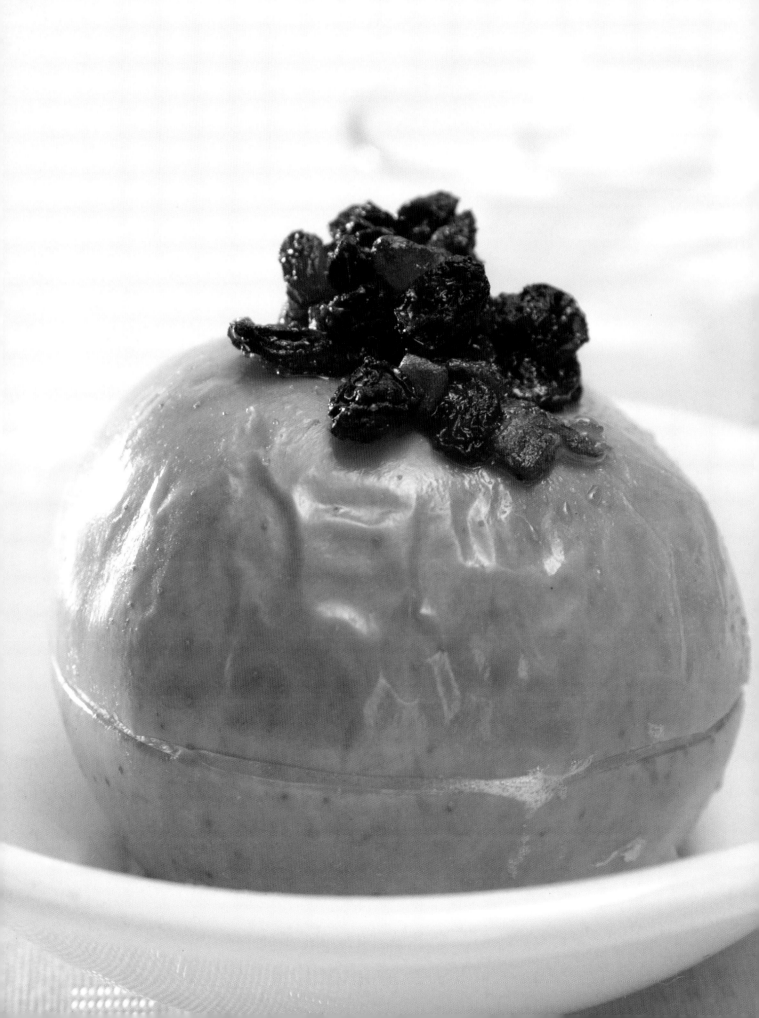

Baked Apples

Family Favourite

These are simple to prepare. The mincemeat is already sweetened, so do not be tempted to add extra sugar. Serve with low-fat crème fraîche, or custard made with skimmed milk and only a little sugar (ready-made low-fat custard tends to be very sweet) for a special treat.

Ingredients for 2

**2 small Bramley cooking
   apples or Granny Smith
   dessert apples
4 tsp reduced-fat mincemeat
2 tbsp sultanas or raisins**

Ingredients for 4

**4 small Bramley cooking
   apples or Granny Smith
   dessert apples
3 tbsp reduced-fat
   mincemeat
4 tbsp sultanas or raisins**

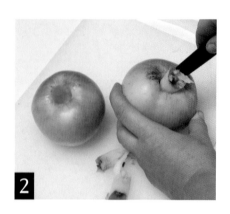

1 Preheat the oven to 180°C/350°F/gas mark 4.

2 Using a potato peeler or apple corer, remove the cores from the apples.

3 Cut a slit in the skin around the centre of each apple. This stops the apple exploding as it cooks.

4 Mix together the mincemeat and dried fruit. Push into the centre of the apple packing down tightly. Place the apples on a baking sheet.

5 Bake the apples for 30–45 minutes until very tender. Allow to stand for 10 minutes before serving.

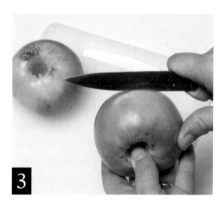

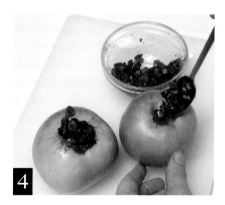

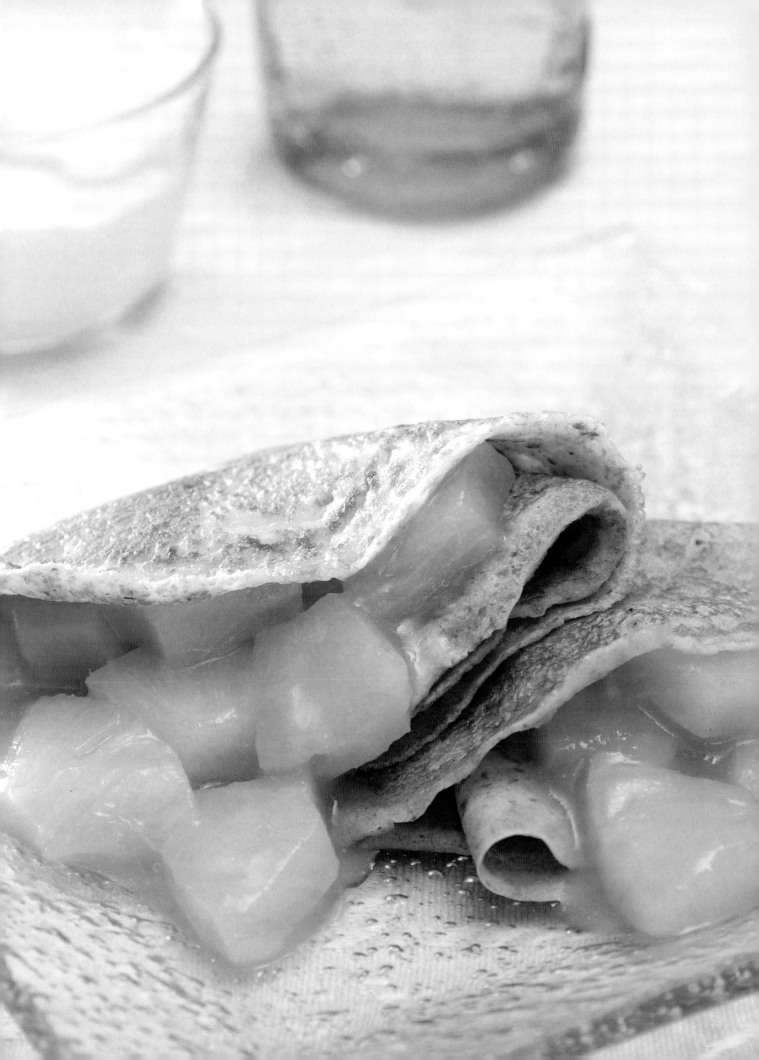

Pineapple Pancakes

These pancakes are very tasty and easy to make. The fruit will count towards your five-a-day.

Makes 6 pancakes

25g/1oz plain flour
25g/1oz plain wholemeal
　flour
1 egg
150ml/¼pt skimmed milk
a little oil for frying

Filling:

200g/7oz can pineapple
　chunks in natural juice
1 tsp sunflower oil
1 tsp light muscovado sugar
1 tsp cornflour
1 tbsp brandy

Makes 12 pancakes

50g/2oz plain flour
50g/2oz plain wholemeal
　flour
2 eggs
300ml/½pt skimmed milk
a little oil for frying

Filling:

400g/14oz can pineapple
　chunks in natural juice
2 tsp sunflower oil
2 tsp light muscovado sugar
2 tsp cornflour
2 tbsp brandy

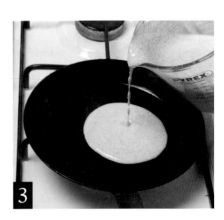

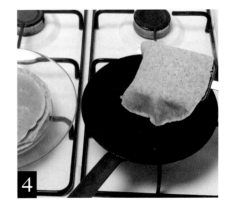

1 Place the flours, egg and milk in a food processor or liquidiser and blend until a smooth batter is formed. Allow to stand for 10 minutes.

2 Heat a little of the oil in a heavy-based, 15–18cm/ 6–7in frying pan.

3 Spoon about 3 tbsp of the batter into the pan and tilt to coat the base. Cook for about 1 minute until the underside is golden.

4 Flip over and cook the other side. Slide out of the pan and keep warm. Repeat with the remaining batter to make 4 (8) pancakes.

5 To keep warm, stack the pancakes on top of each other. Cover with foil and put them in a warm oven or on a plate over a pan of hot water.

6 To make the filling drain the pineapple, reserving the juice. Heat the oil in a small frying pan and fry the pineapple rings for 2–3 minutes each side. Sprinkle over the sugar.

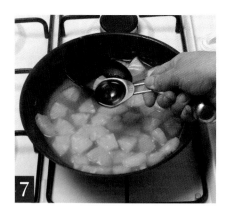

7 Mix the cornflour with a little of the juice. Pour the remaining juice and cornflour mixture into the pan and cook, stirring until thickened slightly. Stir in the brandy.

8 Serve the pancakes folded or rolled with a little of the pineapple filling inside.

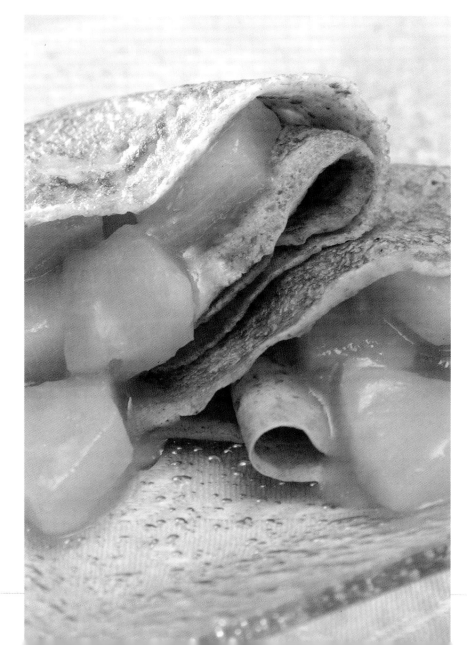

Free-form Apple Pie

Family Favourite

Gram flour is made from chick peas which add soluble fibre to this dish.

Ingredients for 3-4

50g/2oz wholemeal flour
25g/1oz gram flour
40g/1½oz butter or sunflower margarine
about 1 tbsp cold water
1 tbsp ground rice
250g/9oz eating apples
½ tsp fennel seeds
a little egg white
½ tsp demerara or golden granulated sugar

Ingredients for 6-8

100g/4oz wholemeal flour
50g/2oz gram flour
75g/3oz butter or sunflower margarine
about 2 tbsp cold water
2 tbsp ground rice
500g/1lb 2oz eating apples
1 tsp fennel seeds
a little egg white
1 tsp demerara or golden granulated sugar

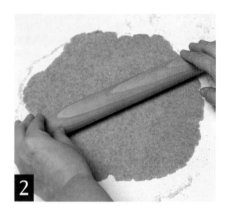

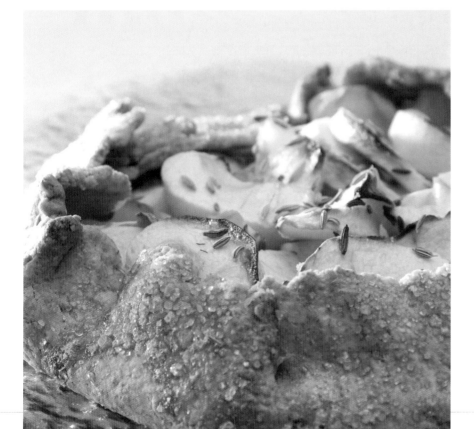

1 Preheat the oven to 200°C/400°F/gas mark 6. Place the flours in a mixing bowl and rub in the fat until the mixture resembles fine breadcrumbs.

2 Add enough water to mix to a soft dough. Roll out the pastry to form a rough circle about 20cm/8in (30cm/12in) across. Place on a lightly greased baking sheet.

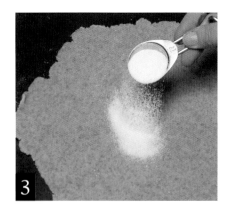

3

3 Sprinkle the ground rice into the centre. This will absorb any moisture from the apples and stop the pastry being soggy.

4 Peel, core and slice the apples and toss with the fennel seeds. Pile into the centre of the pastry.

5 Fold over the edges of the pastry to virtually enclose the apple, leaving just a gap in the centre. Don't worry if the

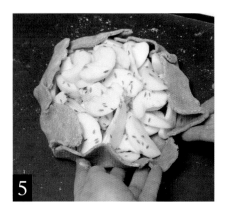

5

pastry cracks or tears a little as this adds to the charm of the dish – just patch it up.

6 Brush the surface of the pastry with a little beaten egg white and sprinkle the sugar over the pastry.

7 Bake for 30–40 minutes until the pastry is crisp and golden.

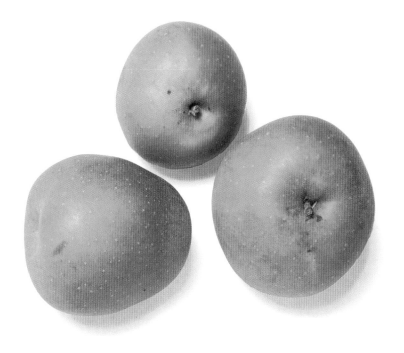

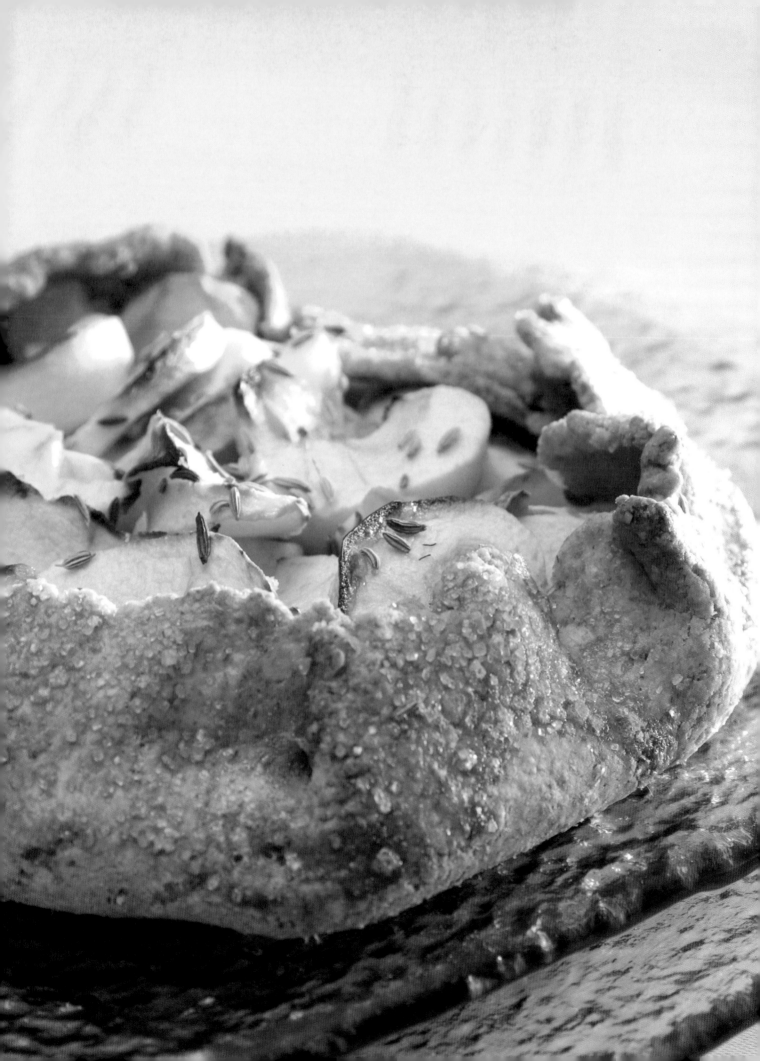

Apricot & Raspberry Fool

Easy Entertaining

Apricots are naturally sweet, so you will not need to add any extra sugar to this creamy dessert.

Ingredients for 2

50g/2oz no-soak dried apricots
50ml/2fl oz boiling water
50g/2oz raspberries
250g/9oz low-fat vanilla or natural yoghurt

Ingredients for 4

100g/4oz no-soak dried apricots
100ml/3½fl oz boiling water
100g/4oz raspberries
500g/1lb 2oz low-fat vanilla or natural yoghurt

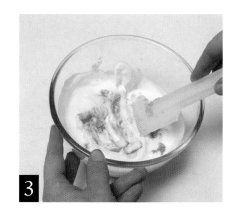

1 Place the apricots in a food processor with the boiling water and blend to form a smooth purée. Allow to cool.

2 Reserve a few raspberries to decorate.

3 Fold the apricot purée into half the yoghurt and the raspberries into the remaining yoghurt.

4 Layer the two yoghurt mixtures in serving glasses. Arrange the reserved raspberries on top and chill for at least 30 minutes before serving.

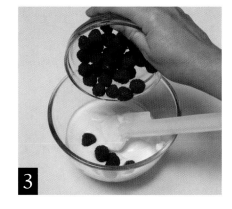

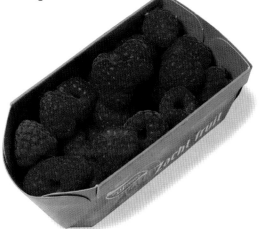

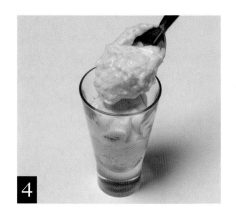

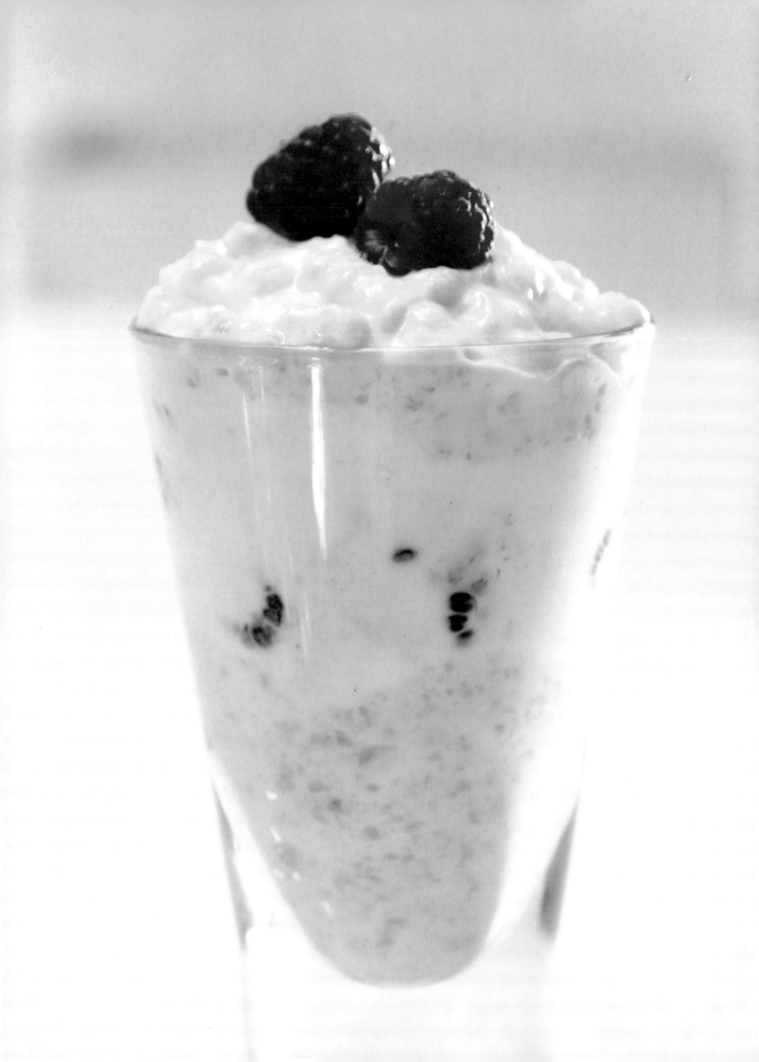

Brown Rice Pudding with Rum Soaked Fruit

You need only a minimum of sugar in this rice dessert as the raisins add sweetness. If you are making it for children, you can soak the raisins in orange juice instead.

Ingredients for 2

50g/2oz raisins or sultanas
1 tbsp rum
50g/2oz short-grain brown rice
200g/7oz can unsweetened evaporated milk
2 tsp light muscovado sugar
pinch of freshly grated nutmeg

Ingredients for 4

100g/4oz raisins or sultanas
2 tbsp rum
100g/4oz short-grain brown rice
400g/14oz can unsweetened evaporated milk
4 tsp light muscovado sugar
pinch of freshly grated nutmeg

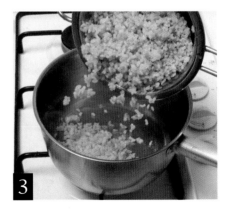

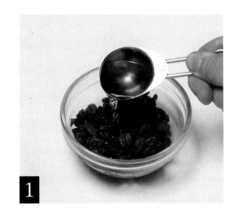

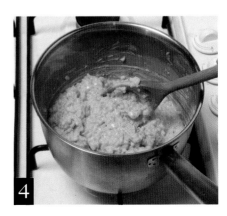

1 Place the fruit in a small bowl, pour over the rum and leave the fruit to soak.

2 Bring a pan of water to the boil, stir in the rice, reduce the heat and simmer gently for 45 minutes until the rice is just tender.

3 When the rice is cooked, drain and return to the pan.

4 Stir in the milk and sugar and cook for about 15 minutes over a low heat until the rice is thick and creamy and most of the milk has been absorbed. Stir frequently to prevent the mixture from burning on the bottom of the pan.

5 Spoon into serving dishes and sprinkle with a little nutmeg. Serve the rum-soaked fruit with the rice puddings.

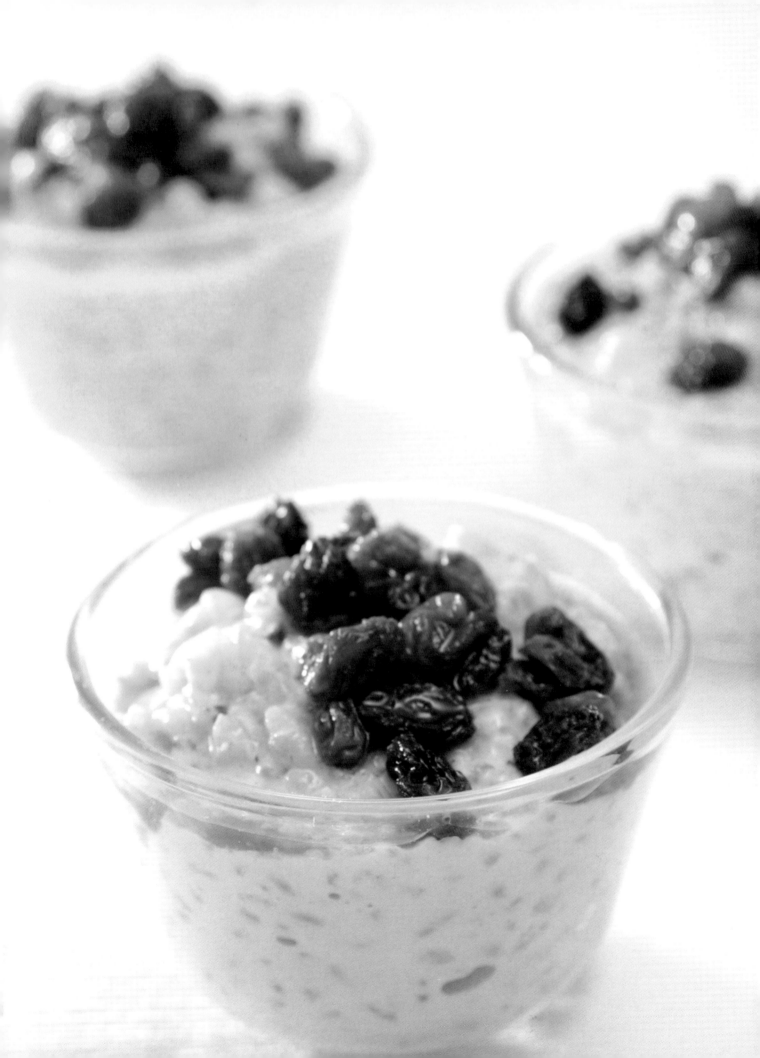

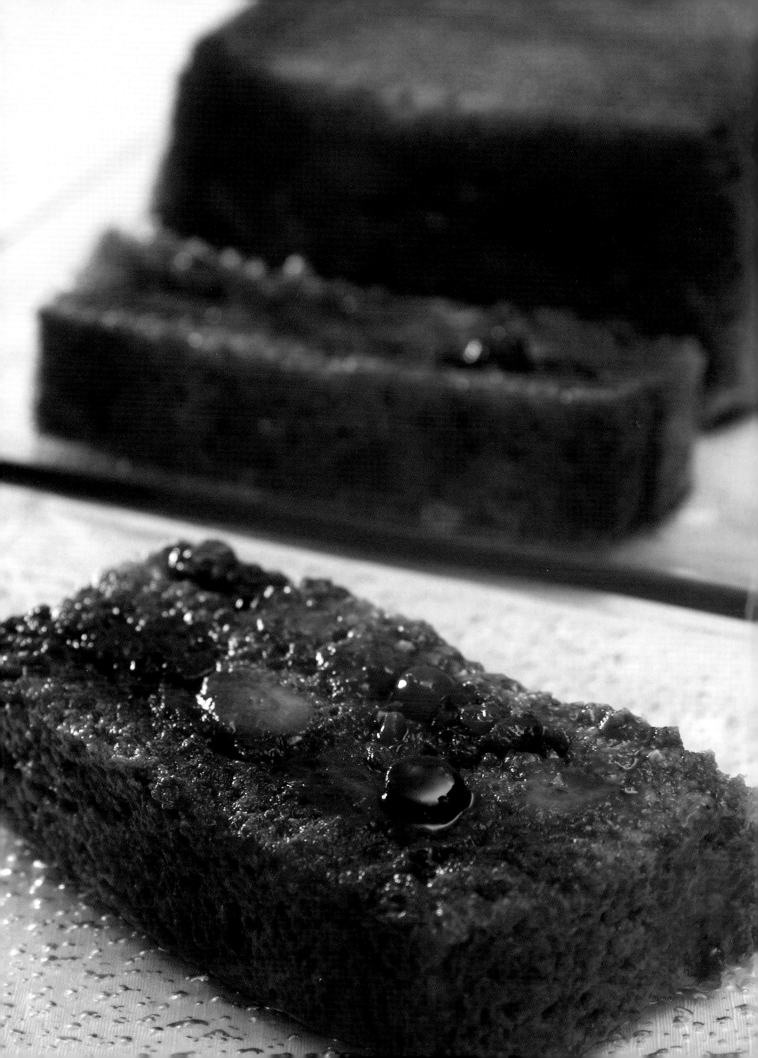

Summer Pudding Loaf

Family Favourite

A perfect summer dessert. Serve with low-fat Greek yoghurt, fromage frais or crème fraîche. You will need to line the tin with cling wrap unless it is non-stick, because the fruit will react with the metal giving the dessert an unpleasant tang.

Serves 8

700g/1½lb mixed soft summer fruits e.g. raspberries, blackberries, strawberries, red and black currants
50g/2oz golden caster sugar or 4 tbsp clear honey
8-10 slices wholemeal bread

1 Line a 900g/2lb loaf tin with cling wrap. Prepare the fruit as necessary, wash and drain well.

2 Place in a saucepan with the sugar or honey and cook over a low heat until the fruits are just tender and the juices begin to run.

3 Remove the crust from the bread and use to line the base and side of the loaf tin. Spoon in half the fruit.

4 Place a layer of bread over the fruit, add the remaining fruit and cover with bread.

5 Cut a thick piece of cardboard the size of the top of the loaf tin. Cover the bread with cling wrap and place the cardboard on top. Weight down with a couple of cans of food and chill overnight.

6 To serve, carefully turn out the pudding on to a serving plate and cut into slices to serve.

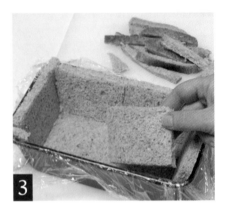

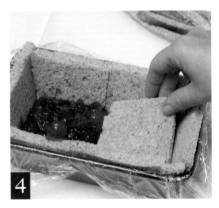

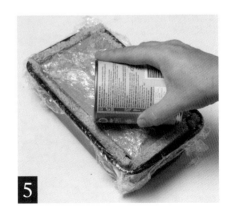

Yoghurt Ice

Ice cream is full of fat, so best saved for special occasions, but a yoghurt ice makes a great alternative that is much lower in fat and calories.

Ingredients for 2

1 small ripe mango
150g/5oz low-fat Greek
    yoghurt
1 tbsp honey
1 small egg white

Ingredients for 4

1 large ripe mango
300g/10½oz low-fat Greek
    yoghurt
2 tbsp honey
1 large egg white

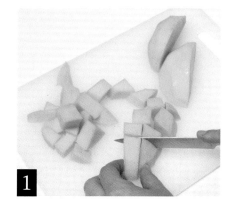

1 Peel and stone the mango, cut into chunks and purée in a food processor.

2 Add the yoghurt and honey and blend.

3 Transfer to a mixing bowl.

4 Whisk the egg whites until standing in soft peaks. Fold into the yoghurt mixture.

5 Pour into a freezer container and freeze for 2 hours, until firm but not solid. Then break up the ice crystals with a fork. Return to the freezer and freeze until firm.

6 Remove from the freezer about 30 minutes before required to soften.

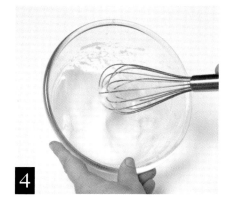

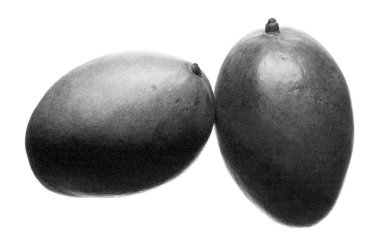

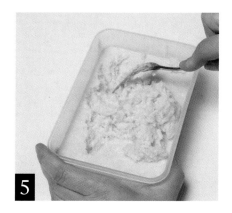

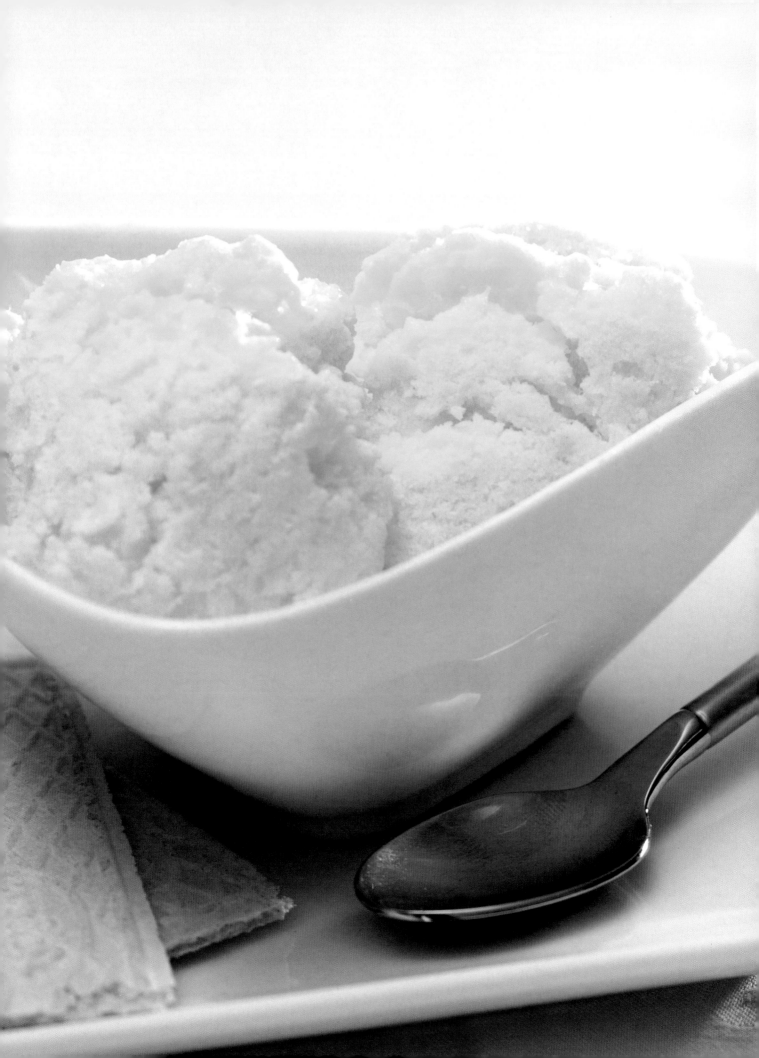

Rhubarb Oat Crumble

Family Favourite

Adding oats to a traditional crumble topping not only improve the texture but adds valuable soluble fibre which releases energy slowly.

Ingredients for 3-4

350g/12oz rhubarb, washed
15g/½oz golden caster sugar
grated zest and juice
¼ orange
1 tsp cornflour

For the topping:

40g/1½oz wholemeal plain flour
25g/1oz butter or sunflower margarine, cut into cubes
40g/1½oz rolled oats
1 tbsp golden caster sugar

Ingredients for 4-6

700g/1½lb rhubarb, washed
25g/1oz golden caster sugar
grated zest and juice
½ orange
2 tsp cornflour

For the topping:

75g/3oz wholemeal plain flour
50g/2oz butter or sunflower margarine, cut into cubes
75g/3oz rolled oats
1 tbsp golden caster sugar

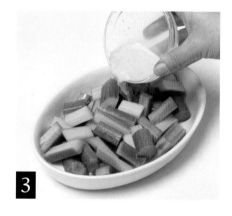

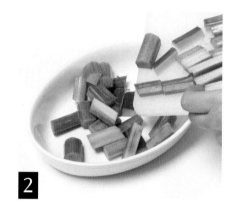

1 Preheat the oven to 200°C/400°F/gas mark 6.

2 Cut the rhubarb into short pieces and place in a shallow pie dish. Add the caster sugar and toss to coat.

3 Combine the orange juice, zest and cornflour and stir into the rhubarb.

4 To make the topping, place the flour in a bowl. Add the butter or margarine and rub in with your fingertips until the mixture resembles coarse breadcrumbs. Stir in the oats and sugar.

5 Sprinkle the topping over the fruit and bake for 35–40 minutes, or until the top is crisp and golden.

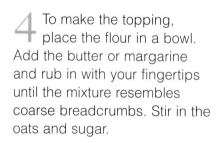

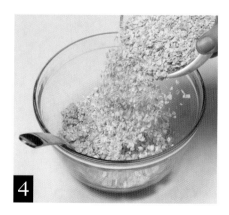

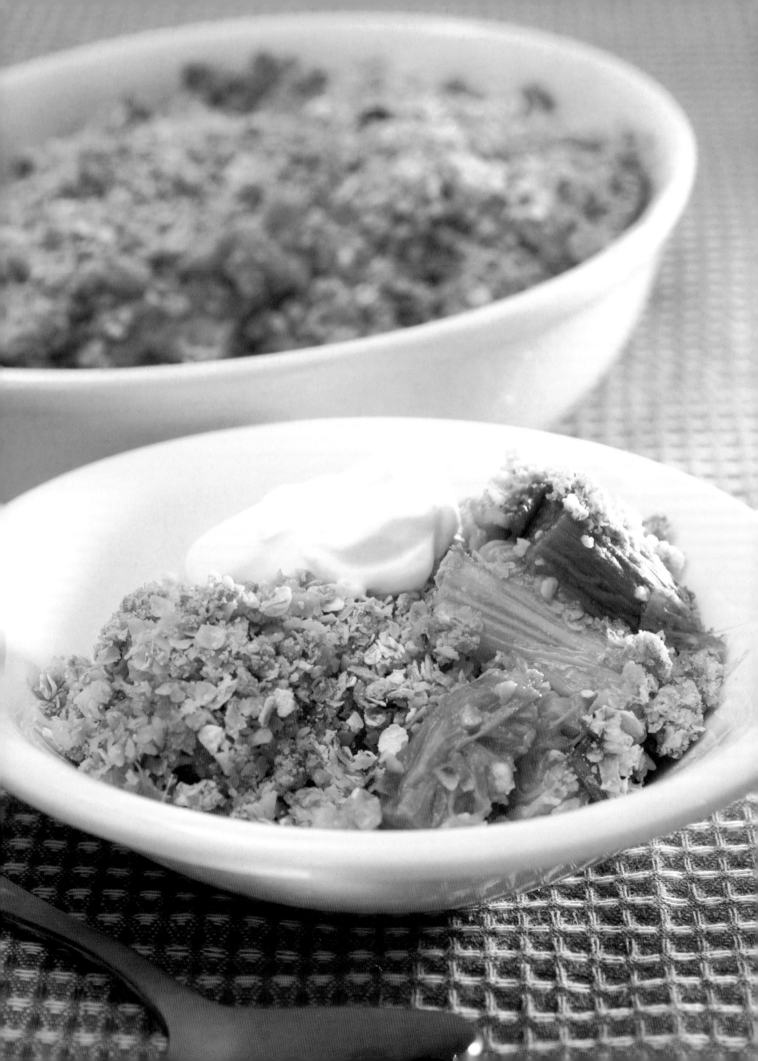

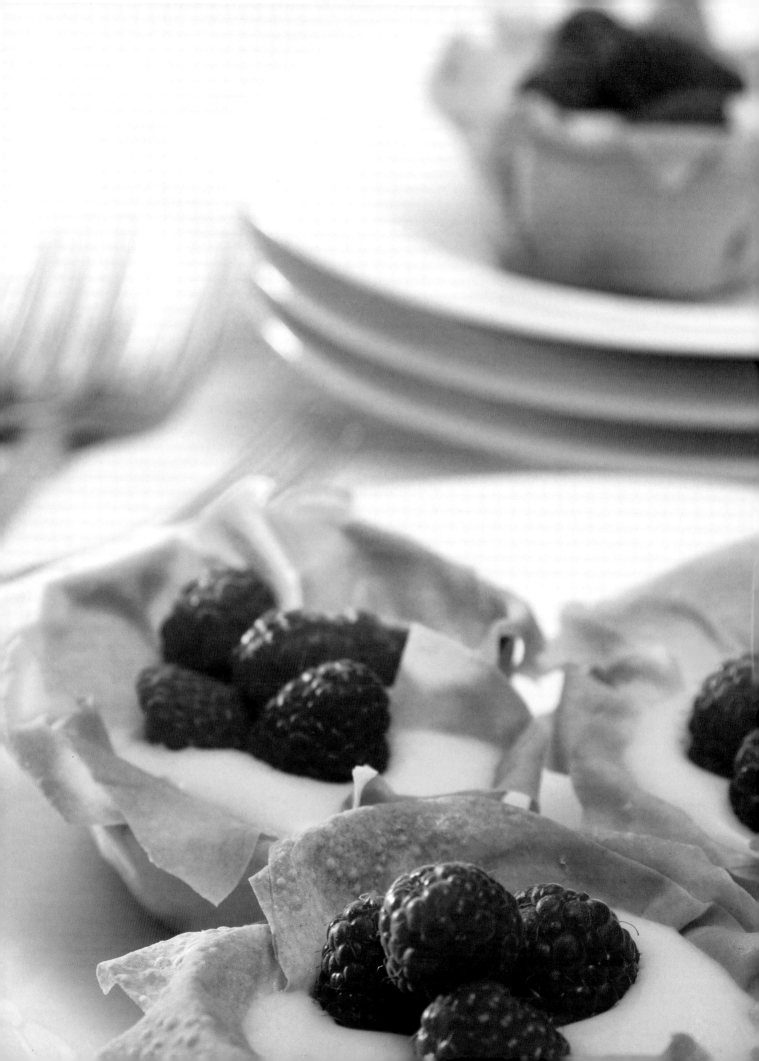

Raspberry Custard Cups

Easy Entertaining

These attractive tarts are low in fat. The pasty cases can be made a few days in advance and stored in an airtight container.

Ingredients for 6

about 2 sheets of filo pastry
about 2 tsp sunflower oil
2 tbsp custard powder
1 tsp golden caster sugar
200ml/7fl oz skimmed milk
75g/3oz fresh raspberries

Ingredients for 12

About 4 sheets of filo pastry
about 4 tsp sunflower oil
4 tsp custard powder
2 tsp golden caster sugar
400ml/14fl oz skimmed milk
175g/6oz fresh raspberries

1 Preheat the oven to 200°C/400°F/gas mark 6.

2 Cut the filo pastry into 18 (36) squares of about 10cm/4in.

3 Brush each square with a little oil and stack 3 squares on top of each other, slightly staggered.

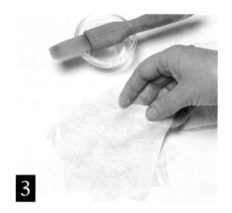

4 Push into a lightly oiled muffin tin to form a pastry cup. Repeat until you have used all the squares and have 6 (12) cups.

5 Bake for 10 minutes or until crisp and golden.

6 Meanwhile, mix together the custard powder, sugar and a little milk to form a smooth paste.

7 Heat the remaining milk until almost boiling. Pour into the custard powder mix, then return to the pan. Cook over a low heat, stirring constantly until thickened.

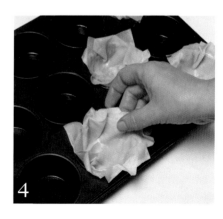

8 Spoon the custard into the filo cups and top with raspberries. Serve immediately. Alternatively allow the custard to cool before filling the cups and serve cold. Fill the cups just before serving

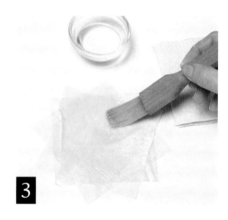

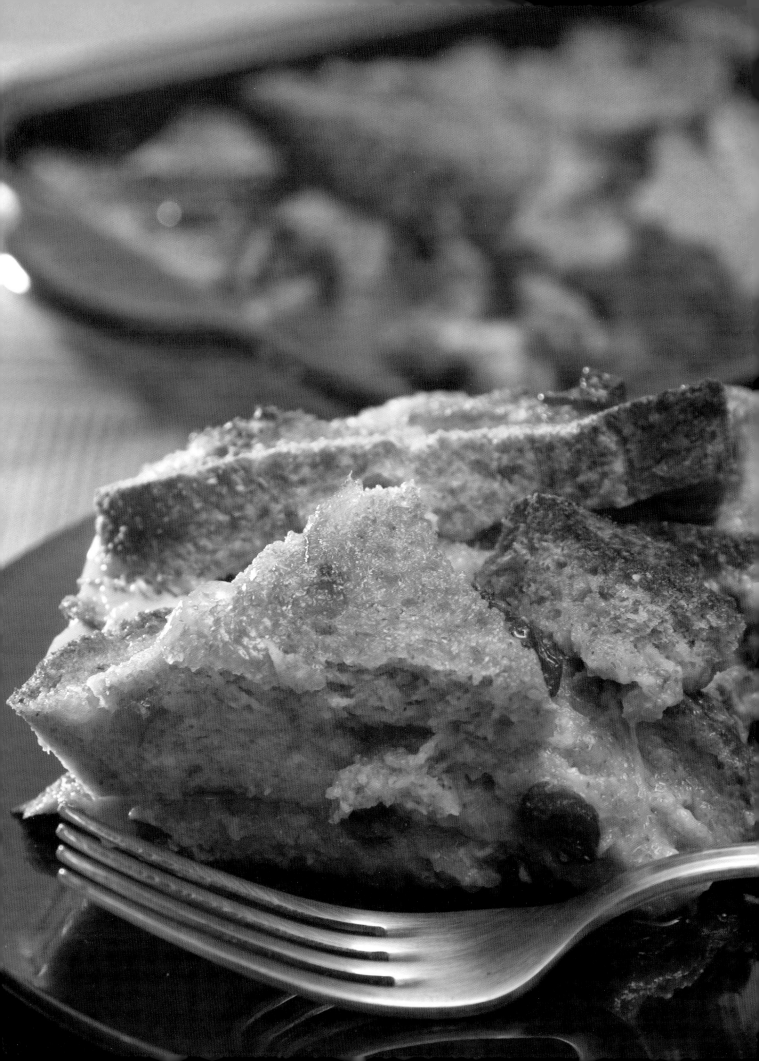

Orange Marmalade Pudding

One Pot

Lower in fat than the standard bread and butter pudding, this version still has loads of flavour and makes a great occasional treat.

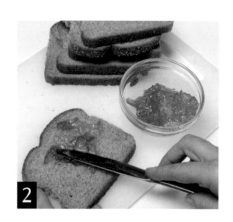

Ingredients for 2

4 slices wholemeal bread
2 tbsp thin shred marmalade
40g/1½oz sultanas
2 small eggs
300ml/½pt skimmed milk
freshly grated nutmeg

Ingredients for 4

6 slices wholemeal bread
4 tbsp thin shred marmalade
75g/3oz sultanas
3 large eggs
600ml/1pt skimmed milk
freshly grated nutmeg

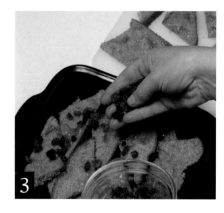

1 Lightly oil a shallow ovenproof dish.

2 Spread the bread with marmalade and cut into quarters. Place a layer of bread in the dish and sprinkle with half the sultanas.

3 Repeat the layers and finish with a layer of bread

4 Beat together the eggs and milk until well combined. Pour over the bread and allow to stand for 20 minutes so that the milk soaks into the bread.

5 Preheat the oven to 180°C/350°F/gas mark 4.

6 Sprinkle with nutmeg. Bake for 45 minutes or until set, risen and golden.

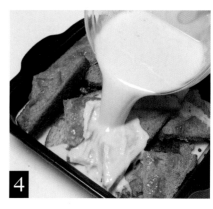

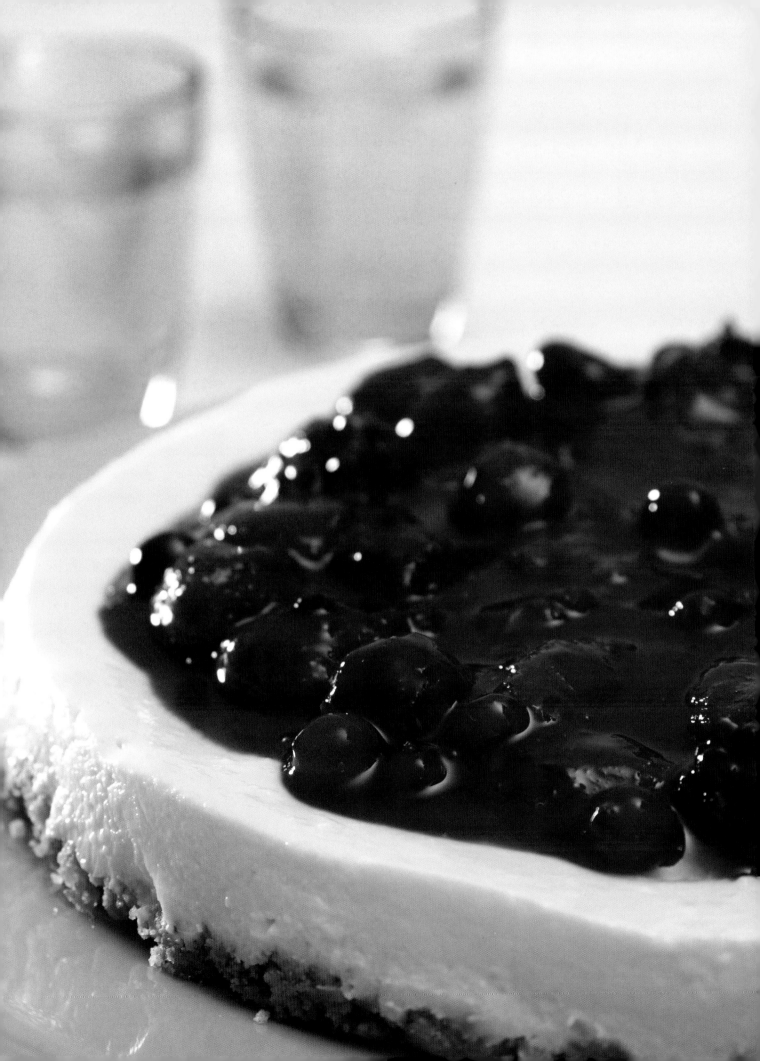

Reduced-fat Cheesecake

Family Favourite

I have reduced the sugar and fat of this cheesecake dramatically, so it makes a healthier option than a traditional cheesecake. Nonetheless it should only be an occasional treat.

Serves 8 to 10

50g/2oz reduced-fat spread
150g/5oz reduced-fat digestive biscuits, crushed
400g/14oz low-fat cream cheese
40g/1½oz golden caster sugar
150g/5oz low-fat Greek yoghurt
2 tsp gelatine
250g/9oz frozen summer fruit, thawed
2 tbsp orange juice
1 tbsp clear honey
1 tbsp cornflour

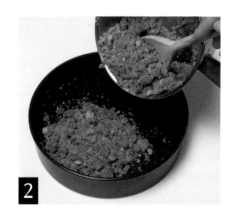

1 Lightly oil and line the base of a 20cm/8in loose-bottomed cake tin.

2 Melt the low-fat spread and stir in the crushed biscuits, mix well and press into the bottom of the prepared cake tin. Chill.

3 Beat together the cheese and sugar, then stir in the yoghurt.

4 Place 2 tbsp water in a small dish and sprinkle the gelatine over the top. Allow the gelatine to go spongy. Dissolve it by standing the bowl in a pan of hot water or in the microwave for 15–20 seconds, stir well, then stir into the cheese mixture.

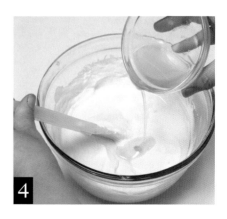

5 Pour over the biscuit base and chill until set.

6 Place the fruit in a small pan with the orange juice and honey. Cook gently until the juices begin to run.

7 Mix the cornflour with 1 tbsp water and stir into the pan. Heat gently, stirring until sauce thickens.

8 Allow to cool, covered with a piece of wetted greaseproof paper (this prevents a skin forming). Spoon over the cheesecake base.

9 Chill until required. Serve cut into wedges

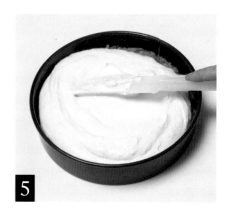

Apple Raisin Cake

Freezer Friendly

This cake is fabulous served as a hot dessert. The fruit adds sweetness allowing the sugar content of the cake to be reduced.

Serves 12

100ml/3½fl oz apple juice
100g/4oz raisins
100g/4oz butter or sunflower margarine
100g/4oz light muscovado sugar
3 eggs
225g/8oz self-raising flour
100g/4oz plain wholemeal flour
½ tsp baking powder
2 small eating apples

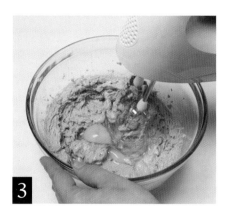

1 Heat the apple juice with the raisins in a small pan until just simmering. Remove from the heat and allow to cool.

2 Preheat the oven to 180°C/350°F/gas mark 4. Lightly oil and line the base of a 23cm/9in square cake tin.

3 Beat together the fat and muscovado sugar until very light and fluffy. Beat in the eggs one at a time, beating well after each addition.

4 Mix together the flours and baking powder, then fold half into the cake mixture.

5 Fold in the soaked raisins and apple juice. Fold in the remaining flour.

6 Peel, core and chop the apples, fold into the cake mixture.

7 Pour into the prepared cake tin and level the top.

8 Bake for 40 minutes until well risen and springy to the touch. Remove from the oven and allow to cool in the tin. Serve cut into squares.

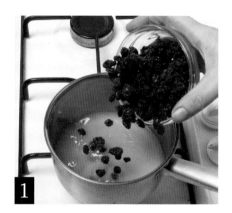

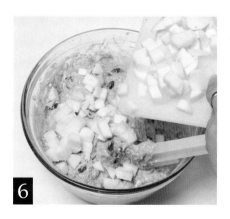

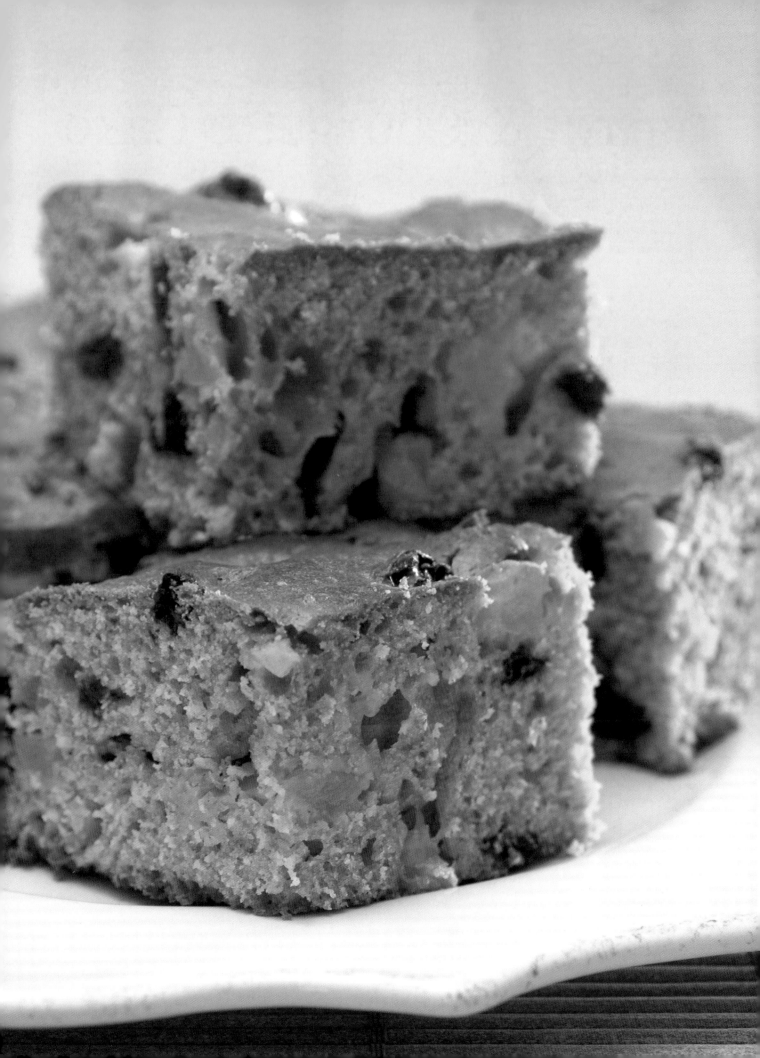

Carrot & Courgette Cake

Carrot cake is well known, this less familiar cake is just as delicious and makes a great teatime treat.

Serves 12

2 eggs
100g/4oz golden caster sugar
1 tsp vanilla essence
225g/8oz carrots, finely grated
225g/8oz courgettes, grated
100ml/3½fl oz sunflower oil
50g/2oz pecan nuts, chopped
100g/4oz plain wholemeal flour
50g/2oz plain flour
1 tsp baking powder
12 pecan halves to decorate

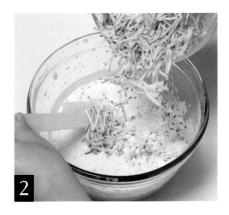

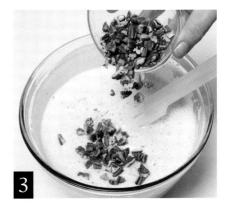

1 Preheat the oven to 180°C/350°F/gas mark 4. Lightly oil a 23cm/9in round loose-bottomed cake tin.

2 Beat the eggs and sugar together until light and fluffy. Stir in the vanilla essence, carrots, courgettes and oil.

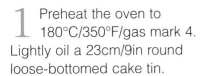

3 Fold in the chopped nuts, flours and baking powder.

4 Pour into the prepared tin and arrange the pecan halves on top.

5 Bake for 40 minutes or until springy to the touch.

6 Serve cut into wedges.

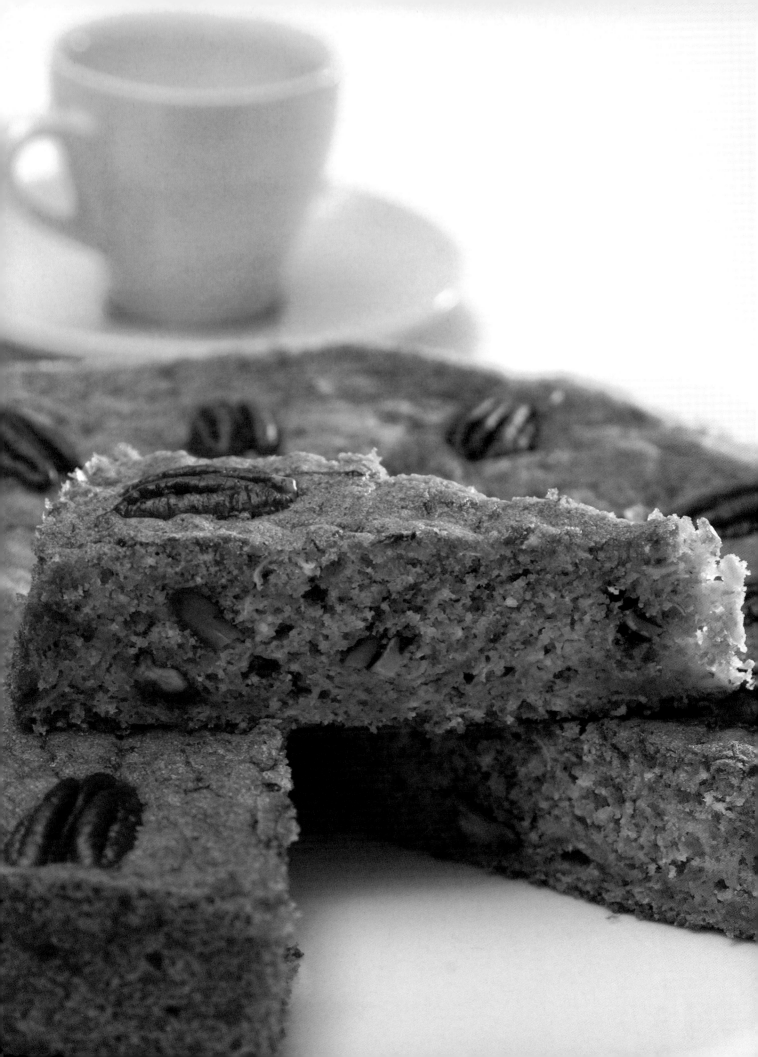

Malt Bread

Freezer Friendly

This loaf is suitable for a midday snack. It can be served plain or spread with a little butter or margarine, but make sure it is only a little and only one slice! The loaf freezes well.

Makes 12 slices

225g/8oz plain flour
225g/8oz plain wholemeal flour
2 tsp baking powder
175g/6oz mixed dried fruit
1 tbsp honey
1 tbsp molasses or black treacle
3 tbsp malt extract
3 tbsp sunflower oil
450ml/¾pt skimmed milk

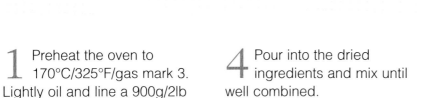

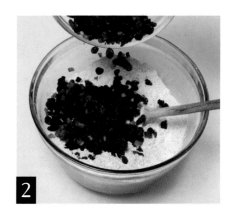

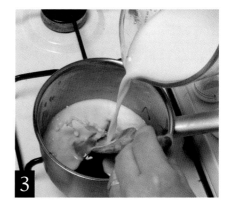

1 Preheat the oven to 170°C/325°F/gas mark 3. Lightly oil and line a 900g/2lb loaf tin.

2 Mix together the flours and baking powder in a large mixing bowl, then stir in the dried fruit.

3 Place all the remaining ingredients except the milk in a small pan and heat gently, stirring until well combined. Remove from the heat and stir in the milk.

4 Pour into the dried ingredients and mix until well combined.

5 Spoon into the prepared tin and bake for about 1¼ hours or until a skewer inserted into the centre comes out clean.

6 Allow to cool in the tin for 5 minutes before turning out on a wire rack to cool completely

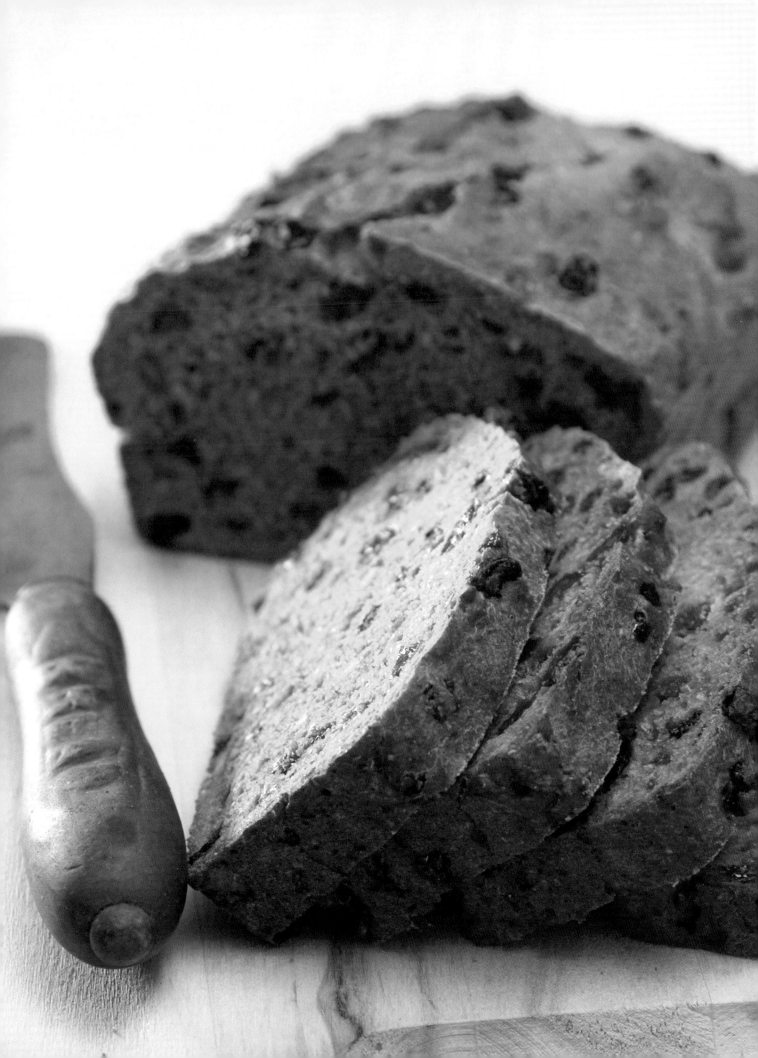

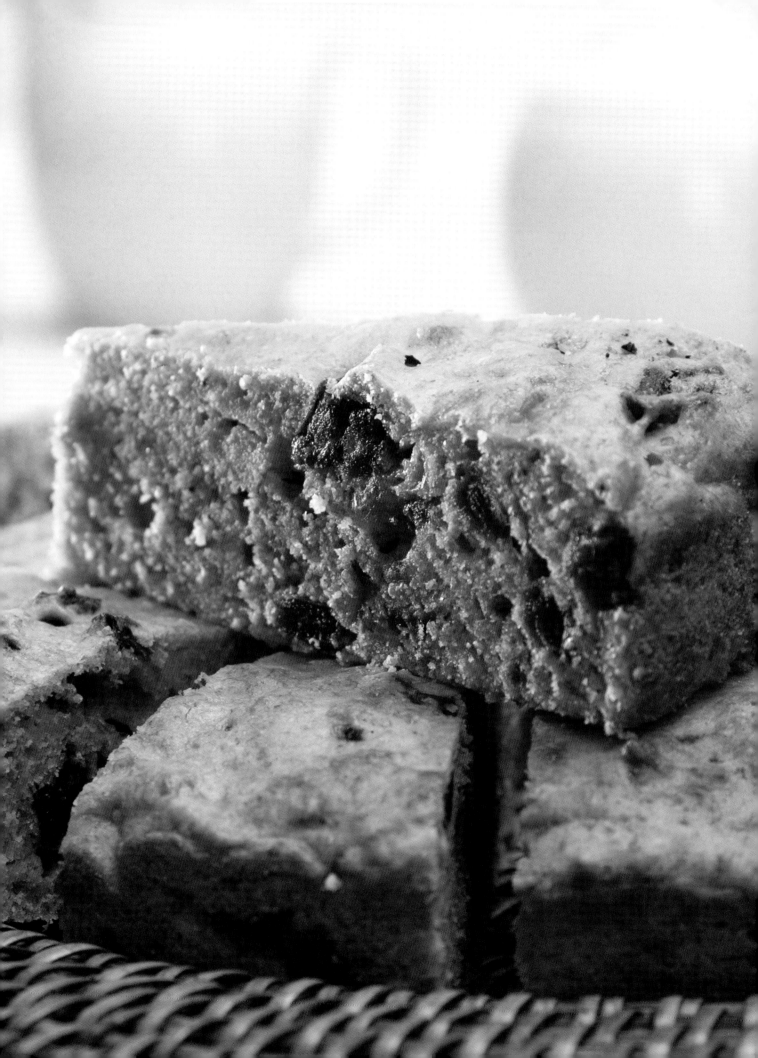

Banana & Date Cake

Rich, moist and fruity. You could add a small slice of this cake to lunch or eat it as a mid-afternoon snack.

Serves 8 to 10

4 medium bananas, about 350g/12oz weight after peeling
225g/8oz plain flour
100g/4oz plain wholemeal flour
1 tsp baking powder
100ml/3½fl oz sunflower oil
75g/3oz light muscovado sugar
3 eggs
150g/5oz pitted dates, chopped

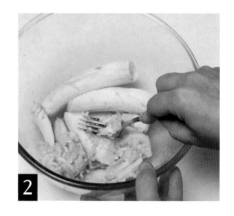

1 Preheat the oven to 190°C/375°F/gas mark 5. Lightly oil a 23cm/9in round cake tin.

2 Mash the bananas with a fork in a large mixing bowl.

3 Add all the remaining ingredients except the dates and beat until smooth.

4 Stir in the dates.

5 Spoon into the prepared tin and bake for about 45 minutes or until springy to the touch.

6 Allow to cool in the pan for 5 minutes, before transferring to a wire rack to cool completely.

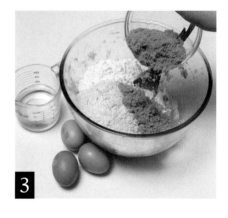

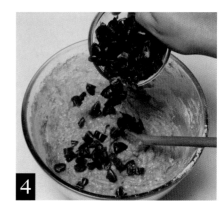

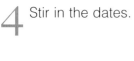

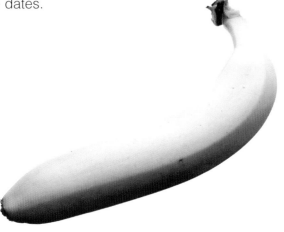

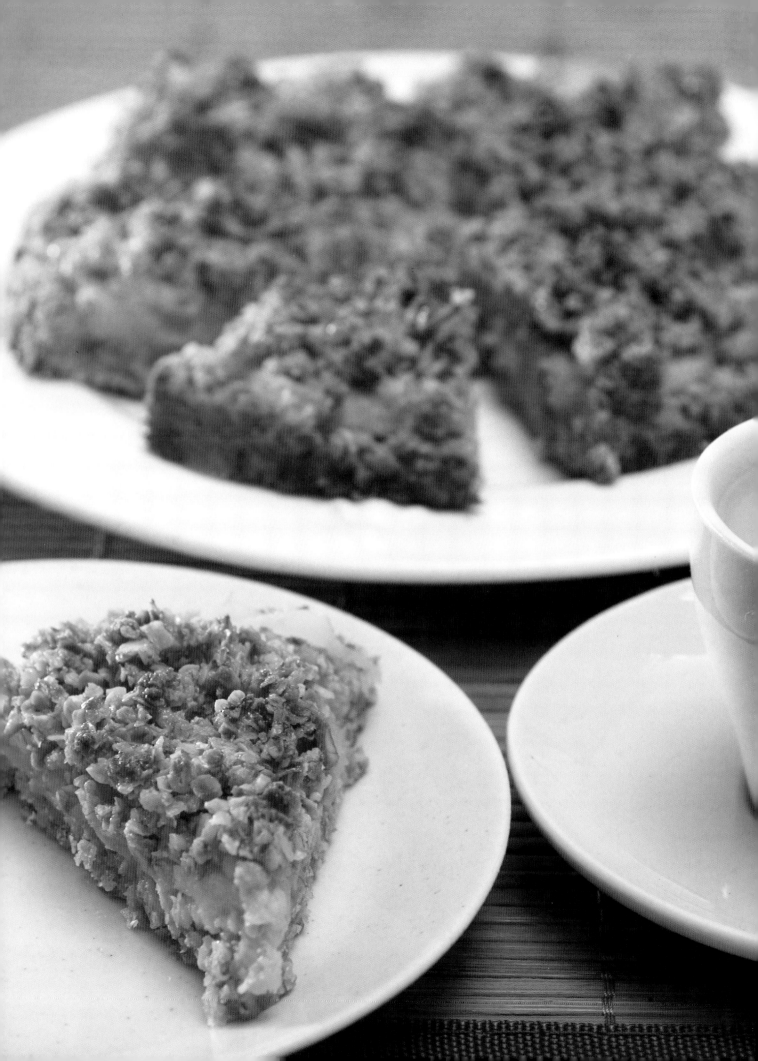

Banana Apple Jacks

Flapjacks with a fruity filling – bliss! If you don't like the flavour of honey, use some date syrup, available from healthfood shops, instead.

Makes about 10

100g/4oz butter or sunflower margarine
50g/2oz light muscovado sugar
4 tbsp clear honey
225g/8oz rolled oats
2 tbsp sunflower seeds

Filling:

225g/8oz eating apples, peeled and sliced
1 tbsp orange juice
1 banana

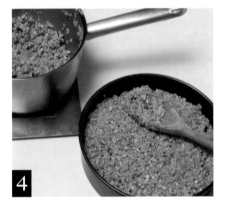

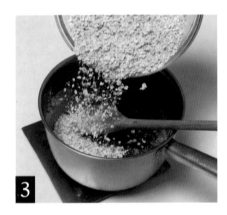

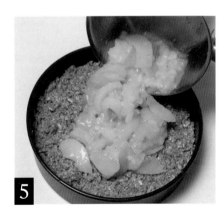

1 Preheat the oven to 170°C/325°F/gas mark 3. Lightly grease a 20cm/8in round, loose-bottom cake tin.

2 Place the butter or margarine, sugar and honey in a saucepan and heat gently, stirring until the fat melts and the sugar dissolves. Remove from the heat.

3 Stir in the oats and sunflower seeds until well combined.

4 Press about two-thirds into the prepared tin and flatten with the spoon.

5 Place the apple and orange juice in a small saucepan and cook, covered, over a low heat for 10 minutes until soft. Mash the banana and stir in. Spread the fruit mix over the oats.

6 Carefully spread the remaining oat mixture over the fruit. Bake for 30–35 minutes until golden.

7 Allow to cool in the tin for 5 minutes before cutting into bars. The bars will be crumbly at first but will harden on cooling.

Orange Oat Muffins

Freezer Friendly

These home-made muffins have a much lower sugar content than most cakes, making then ideal for a snack or even a tasty start to the day served with a small glass of fresh orange juice. They can be frozen and then reheated from frozen at 180°C/350°F/gas mark 4 for 10 minutes.

Ingredients for 12

175g/6oz plain wholemeal flour
50g/2oz plain flour
2 tsp baking powder
100g/4oz rolled oats
4 tbsp golden caster sugar
2 large eggs
150ml/¼pt skimmed milk
150ml/¼pt orange juice
3 tbsp sunflower oil
grated zest ½ orange

1 Preheat the oven to 200°C/400°F/gas mark 6. Line 12 muffin cups with paper cases or greaseproof paper.

2 Combine the flours, baking powder, oats and sugar together in a mixing bowl.

3 In a small bowl, whisk together all the remaining ingredients.

4 Pour the liquid ingredients into the dried ingredients and stir until just moistened. Do not over-beat – the mixture should be lumpy.

5 Spoon into the muffin cases and bake for 15–20 minutes until risen and golden. Serve warm.

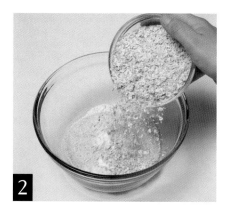

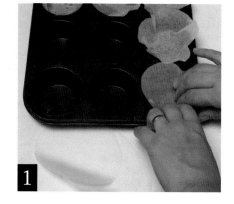

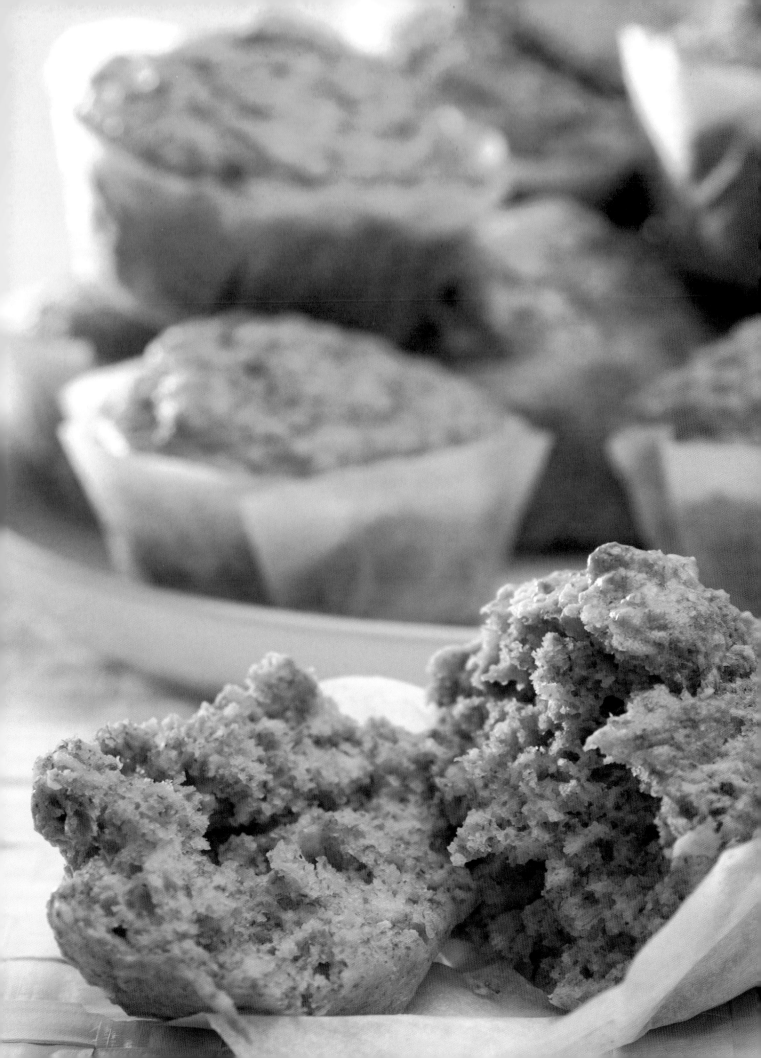

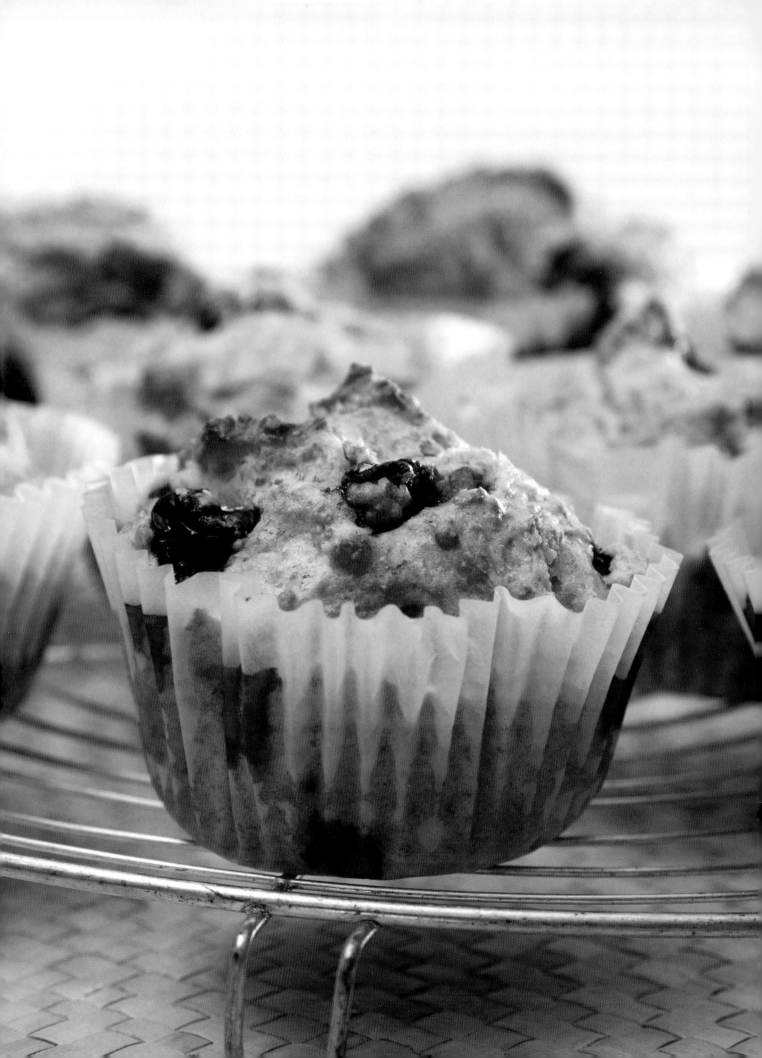

Blueberry & Walnut Muffins

Freezer Friendly

These muffins make a good snack for between meals, and I have also served them for breakfast. They are best served warm and very fresh, so freeze any that are not required that day. Defrost as for Orange Oat Muffins (see page 206) and reheat in a warm oven.

Ingredients for 12

150g/5oz plain flour
150g/5oz plain wholemeal flour
40g/1½oz golden caster sugar
1 tbsp baking powder
75g/3oz walnuts, chopped
125g/4½oz blueberries
150ml/5fl oz low-fat fromage frais
1 egg
150ml/¼pt skimmed milk
3 tbsp sunflower oil
grated zest and juice of ½ lemon

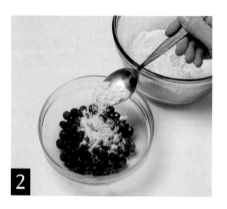

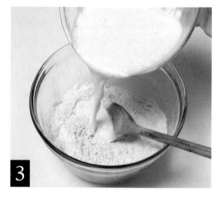

1 Preheat the oven to 200°C/400°F/gas mark 6. Line a 12-cup muffin pan with paper muffin cases or greaseproof paper.

2 Combine the flours, sugar, baking powder and walnuts in a medium bowl. Toss the blueberries with 3 tablespoons of the flour mixture in a small bowl until well coated.

3 Beat the fromage frais, egg, milk, oil, lemon zest and juice together in a large bowl. Add to the flour mixture and mix until moistened.

4 Gently fold in the blueberries. Spoon the batter into the muffin cases. Bake until the muffins are well risen and golden, or until a skewer inserted into the centre comes out clean, about 25 minutes.

5 Place the muffin tin on a wire rack and allow to cool for 5 minutes. Turn the muffins out on to the wire rack. Serve warm or at room temperature.

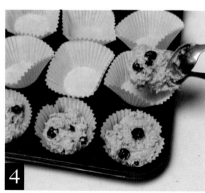

Bread Pudding

Family Favourite

This recipe is great for using up stale bread, and with only a little added sugar it is an ideal teatime treat. Once cool, store in a airtight container for up to 1 week.

Makes 12

350g/12oz bread, cut or torn into cubes (preferably wholemeal)
300ml/½pt milk
150ml/¼pt water
175g/6oz sultanas
1 eating apple, peeled and chopped
2 tbsp golden caster sugar
2 tbsp mixed ground spice
4 tbsp sunflower oil
1 egg, beaten

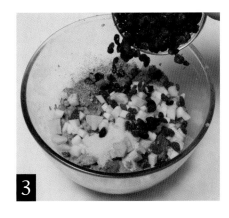

1 Place the bread in a large mixing bowl and pour over the milk and water. Allow the bread to soak up the liquid. This will take longer if the bread is old. Stir occasionally.

2 Preheat the oven to 180°C/350°F/gas mark 4.

3 Stir the sultanas, apple, sugar and spice into the soaked bread and mix until well combined. Beat in the oil and egg.

4 Press into a lightly oiled 23cm/9in square cake tin and bake for 45 minutes.

5 Allow to cool slightly before cutting into 12 squares.

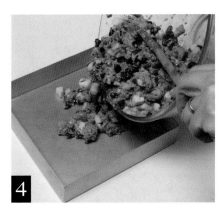

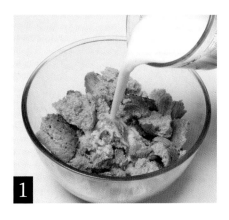

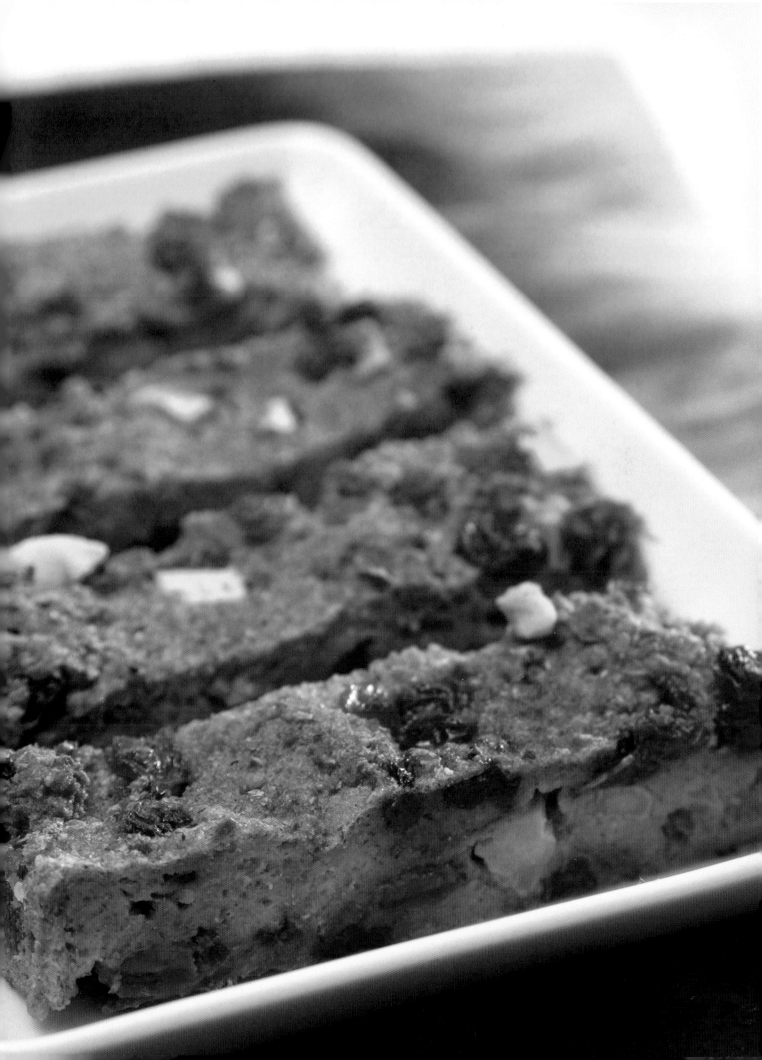

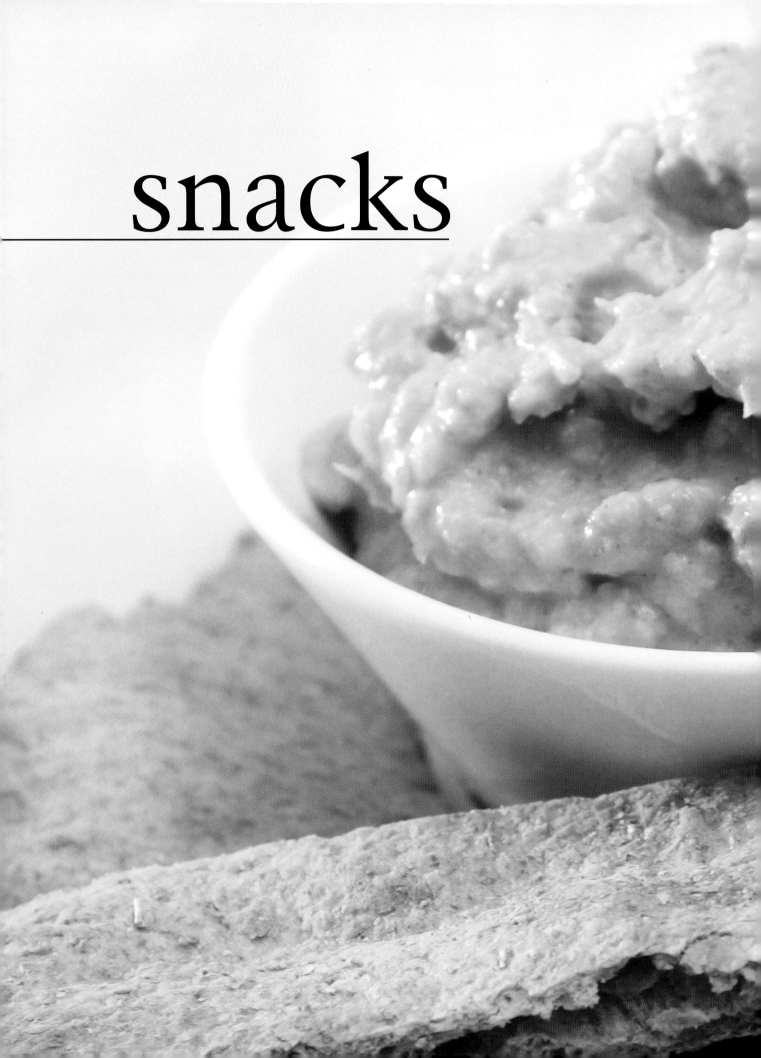

snacks

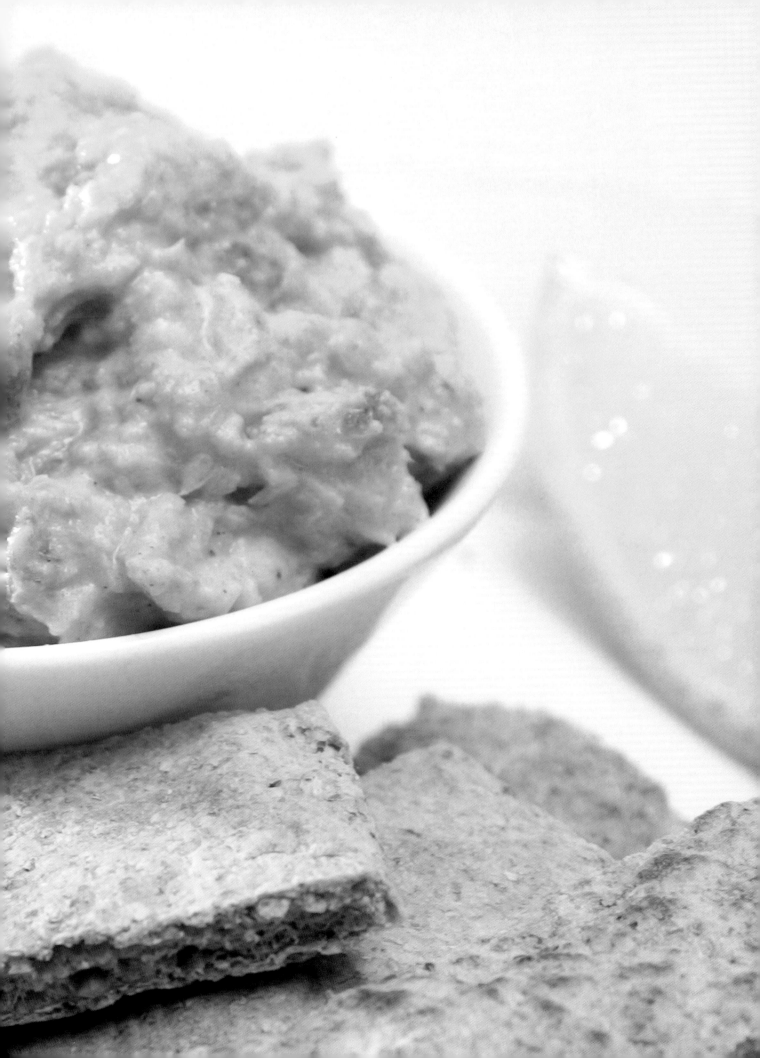

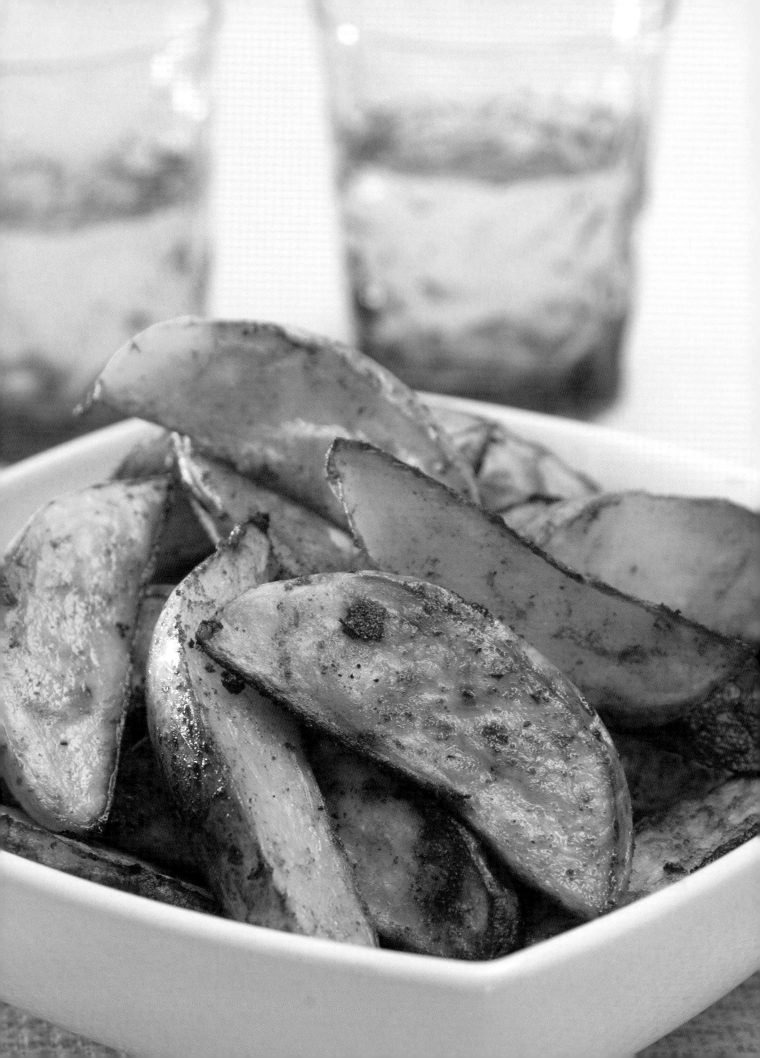

Chilli Oven Wedges

Hot and spicy

Most children love chips, and oven chips are the perfect compromise as they are much lower in fat then normal chips – and just as popular.

Ingredients for 2

**250g/9oz medium floury
  potatoes, washed
1 tbsp sunflower oil
1 tsp chilli sauce
1 tsp paprika**

Ingredients for 4

**500g/1lb 2oz medium floury
  potatoes, washed
2 tbsp sunflower oil
2 tsp chilli sauce
2 tsp paprika**

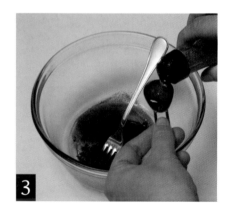

1 Place one or two baking sheets in the oven and preheat the oven to 220°C/425°F/gas mark 7.

2 Cut the potatoes into chunky wedges, rinse in cold water to remove excess starch and pat dry on a clean teacloth or kitchen paper.

3 Combine the oil, chilli sauce and paprika in a large bowl and add the potato wedges. Toss until well coated.

4 Spread out in a single layer on the hot baking sheets. Bake for 25–35 minutes until tender, crisp and golden.

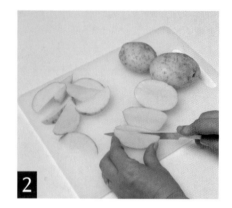

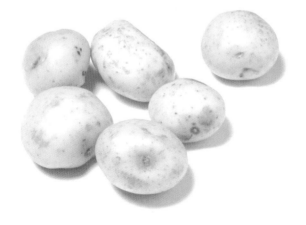

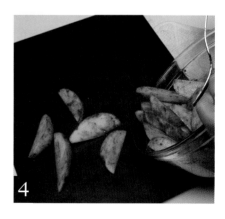

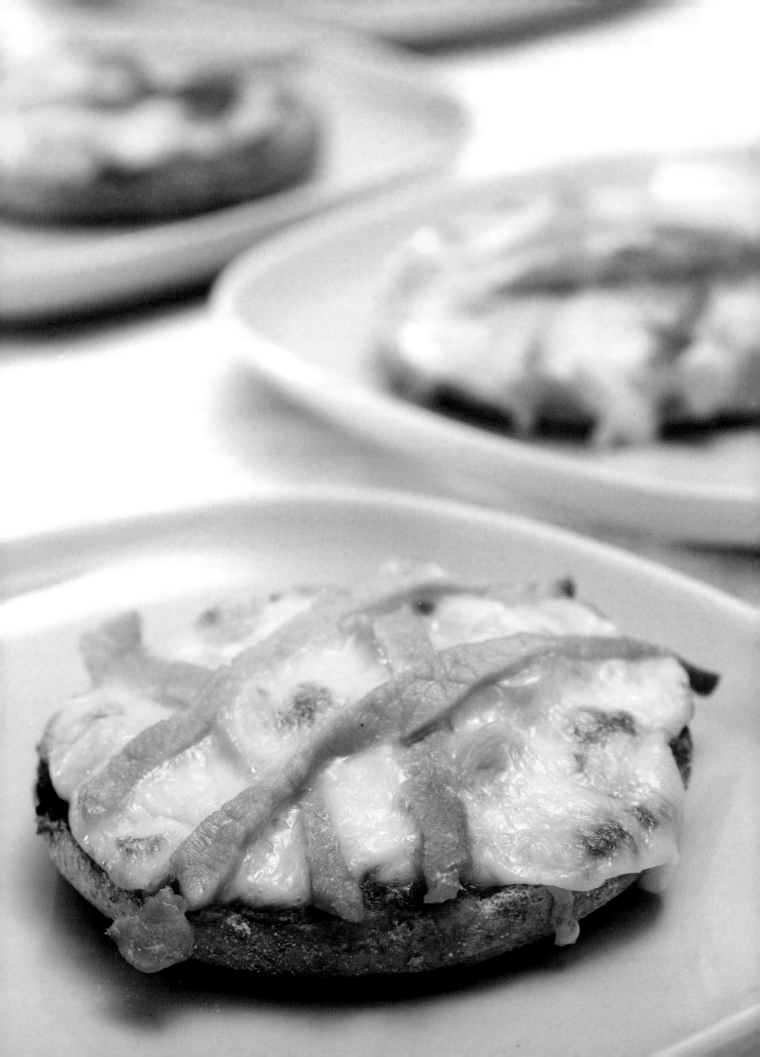

Instant pizzas

Family Favourite

Knock these pizzas up in minutes for a great snack.

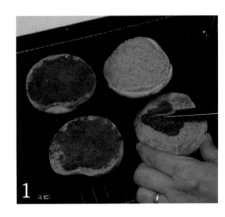

Ingredients for 2

1 wholemeal bread muffin or soft brown roll
2 tbsp tomato purée or tomato pizza topping
2 spring onions, sliced
25g/1oz reduced-fat Cheddar cheese, grated
25g/1oz mozzarella, grated
1 rasher of back bacon, cut into thin strips.

Ingredients for 4

2 wholemeal bread muffins or soft brown rolls
4 tbsp tomato purée or tomato pizza topping
4 spring onions, sliced
50g/2oz reduced-fat Cheddar cheese, grated
50g/2oz mozzarella, grated
2 rashers of back bacon, cut into thin strips.

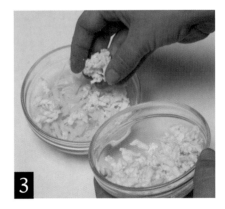

1 Cut the muffins or rolls in half and lightly toast. Spread with the tomato purée or pizza topping.

2 Scatter the spring onions over the top.

3 Mix the cheeses together and pile on top of the pizza.

4 Arrange the bacon in a criss-cross pattern over the pizza.

5 Cook under a hot grill until the cheese begins to brown. Serve immediately.

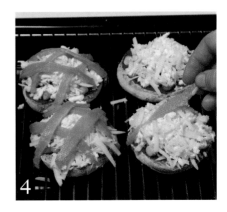

Cheesy Biscuit Nibbles

Freezer Friendly

This is a savoury snack that freezes well. Freeze cooked or uncooked. If cooking from frozen, allow an extra 3–5 minutes cooking time.

Makes 12

50g/2oz reduced-fat red
    Leicester cheese, grated
2 spring onions, chopped
15g/½oz walnuts, chopped
50g/2oz plain wholemeal
    flour
½ tsp whole grain mustard
2 tbsp sunflower oil

Makes 24

100g/4oz reduced-fat red
    Leicester cheese, grated
4 spring onions, chopped
25g/1oz walnuts, chopped
100g/4oz plain wholemeal
    flour
1 tsp whole grain mustard
4 tbsp sunflower oil

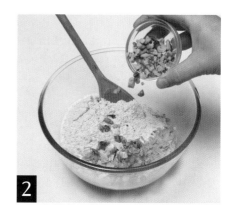

1 Preheat the oven to 190°C/375°F/gas mark 5.

2 Mix together the cheese, onions, walnuts and flour in a mixing bowl.

3 Whisk the mustard into the oil, then add to the dry ingredients and beat until well combined. If the mixture is very dry, add a little water to bind it together.

4 Place spoonfuls of the mixture on to a lightly oiled baking sheet. Flatten slightly with a fork.

5 Bake for about 15 minutes until golden brown. Leave to cool on the tray for 2–3 minutes before transferring to a wire rack to cool completely.

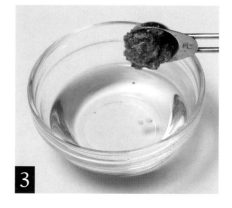

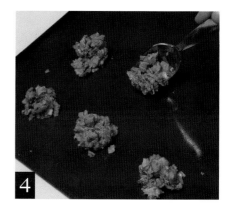

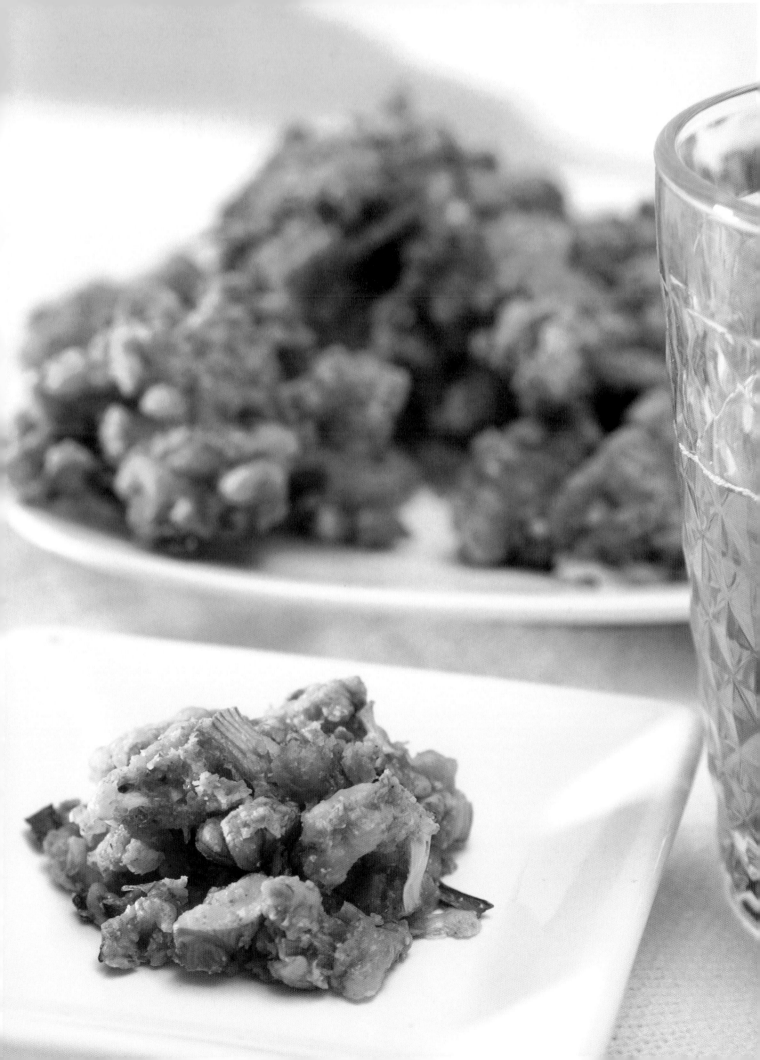

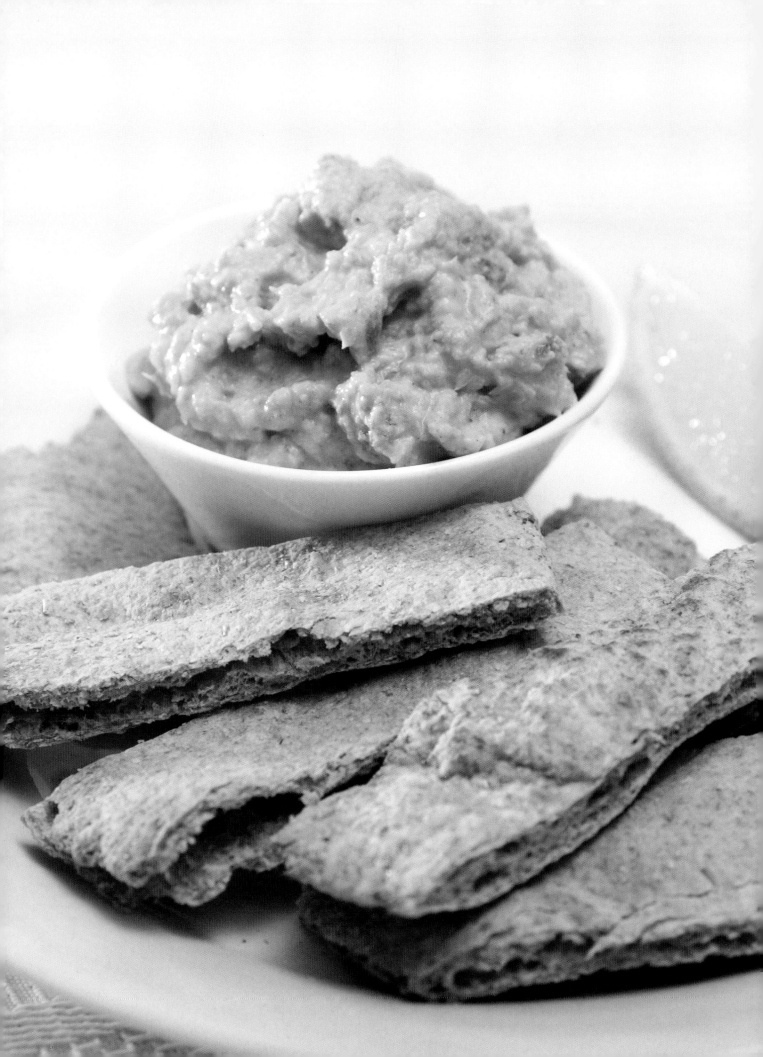

Red Pepper Hummus

Hummus is ideal for snacking. I make my own with the addition of red pepper which gives it extra flavour. Serve with vegetable crudités or toasted wholemeal pitta bread.

Ingredients for 6

1 red pepper
400g/14oz can chick peas, rinsed and drained
2 cloves garlic, crushed
½ tsp ground cumin
½ tsp ground coriander
½ tsp chilli powder
3 tbsp tahini
3 tbsp lemon juice
1 tbsp water

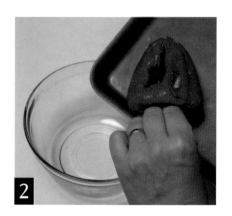

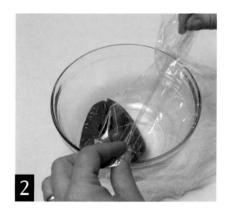

1 Preheat the oven to 200°C/400°F/gas mark 6. Place the pepper on a baking sheet and roast whole for 20–25 minutes, or until skin is blackened.

2 Remove from the oven and place in a bowl. Cover the bowl with cling wrap and allow to cool.

3 Peel the skin away from the pepper and discard. Remove the core and seeds and discard. Place the flesh in a food processor.

4 Place all the remaining ingredients in the food processor and blend until a smooth purée is formed.

5 Spoon into a serving dish and serve. The hummus will keep in the refrigerator for up to 1 week.

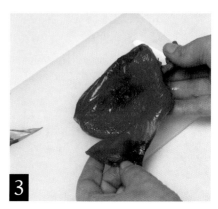

Crab Toasties

Quick and Easy

These spicy, crab-flavoured toasties make a great snack.

Ingredients for 2

1 tsp sunflower oil
2 spring onions, sliced
**½ red chilli, seeded and
  chopped**
**15g/½oz fresh wholemeal
  breadcrumbs**
**50g/2oz canned crab meat,
  drained**
1 tsp skimmed milk
2 slices wholemeal bread
a little beaten egg
salt and pepper
dash of Tabasco sauce

Ingredients for 4

2 tsp sunflower oil
4 spring onions, sliced
**1 red chilli, seeded and
  chopped**
**25g/1oz fresh wholemeal
  breadcrumbs**
**100g/4oz canned crab meat,
  drained**
2 tsp skimmed milk
4 slices wholemeal bread
1 small egg
salt and pepper
dash of Tabasco sauce

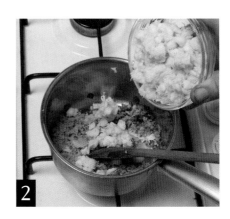

1 Heat the oil in a small pan and stir in the spring onions and chilli. Sauté until softened slightly.

2 Stir in the breadcrumbs, crab meat and milk. Remove from the heat.

3 Lightly toast the bread. Beat the egg until frothy, then stir into the crab mixture.

4 Spread over the toast, making sure that you go right up to the edges or the toast will burn.

5 Place under the grill for a minute or two until just set and golden.

6 Cut in half and serve.

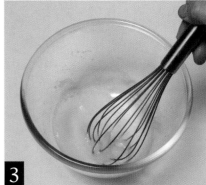

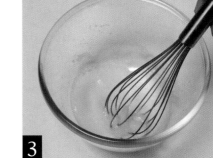

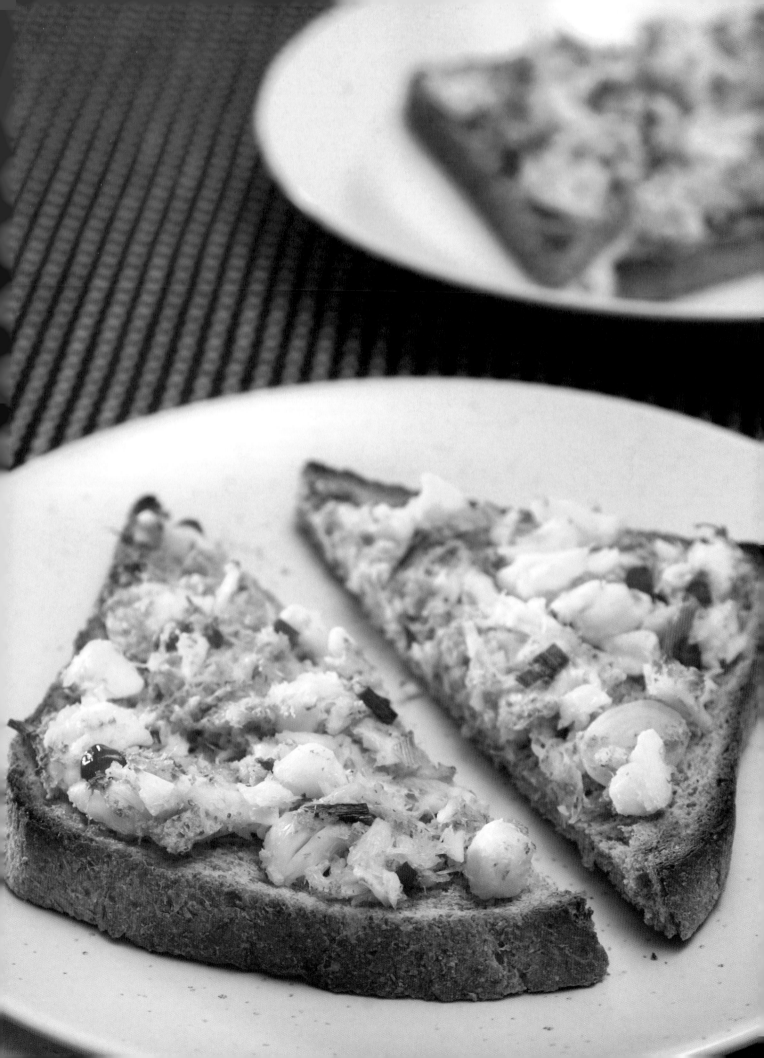

Prawn Toasts

These toasts are usually deep fried, so I have adapted them to give equally good results with much less fat. Serve with drinks or as a tasty snack at any time of the day.

Ingredients for 2

100g/4oz peeled prawns
¼ tsp ground ginger
1 tbsp lightly beaten egg
   white
½ tsp dry sherry
½ tsp cornflour
salt and freshly ground
   black pepper
2 slices wholemeal bread
1 tsp sesame oil
1 tbsp sesame seeds

Ingredients for 4

225g/8oz peeled prawns
½ tsp ground ginger
1 small lightly beaten egg
   white
1 tsp dry sherry
1 tsp cornflour
salt and freshly ground
   black pepper
4 slices wholemeal bread
2 tsp sesame oil
2 tbsp sesame seeds

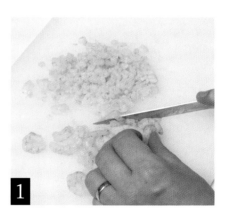

1 Preheat the oven to 190°C/375°F/gas mark 5. Finely chop the prawns and toss with the ginger.

2 Whisk together the egg white, sherry and cornflour with a fork and stir into the prawns. Season well.

3 Lightly toast the bread. Brush one side of the bread with the sesame oil and place oil-side down on a baking sheet.

4 Spread the prawn mixture over the toasts and sprinkle with sesame seeds.

5 Bake for 10–15 minutes until crisp. Serve immediately.

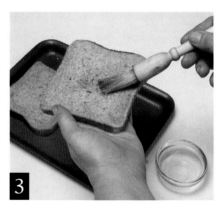

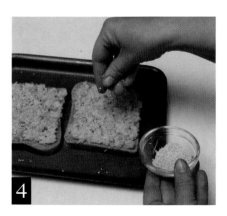

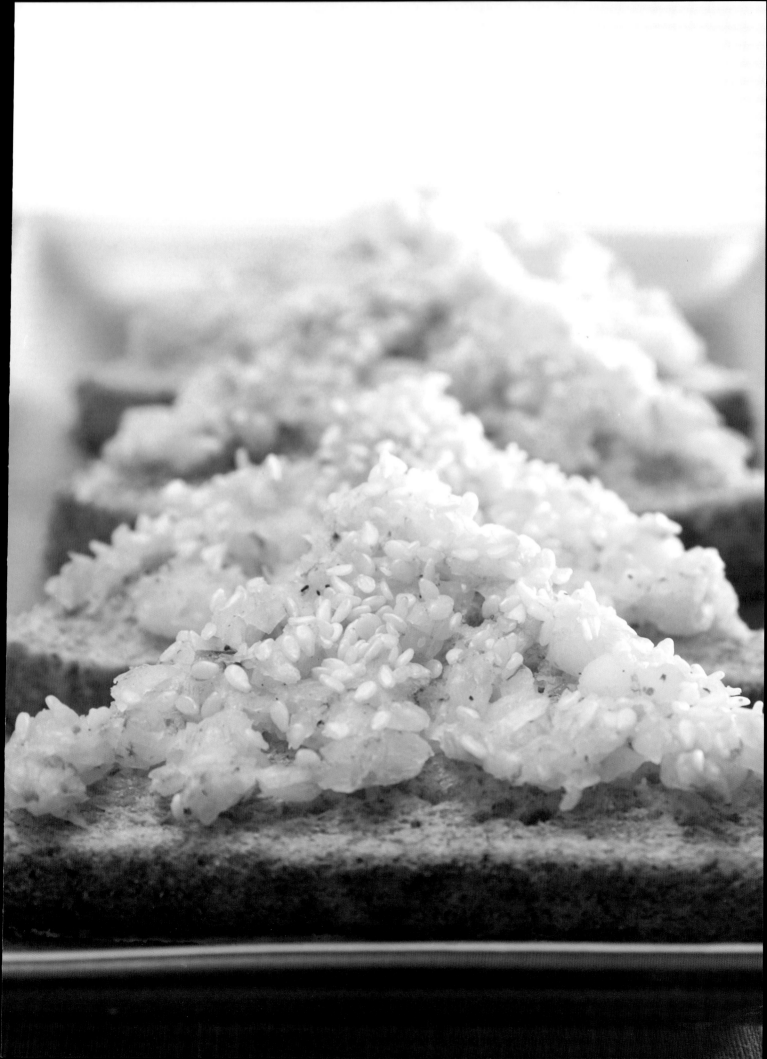

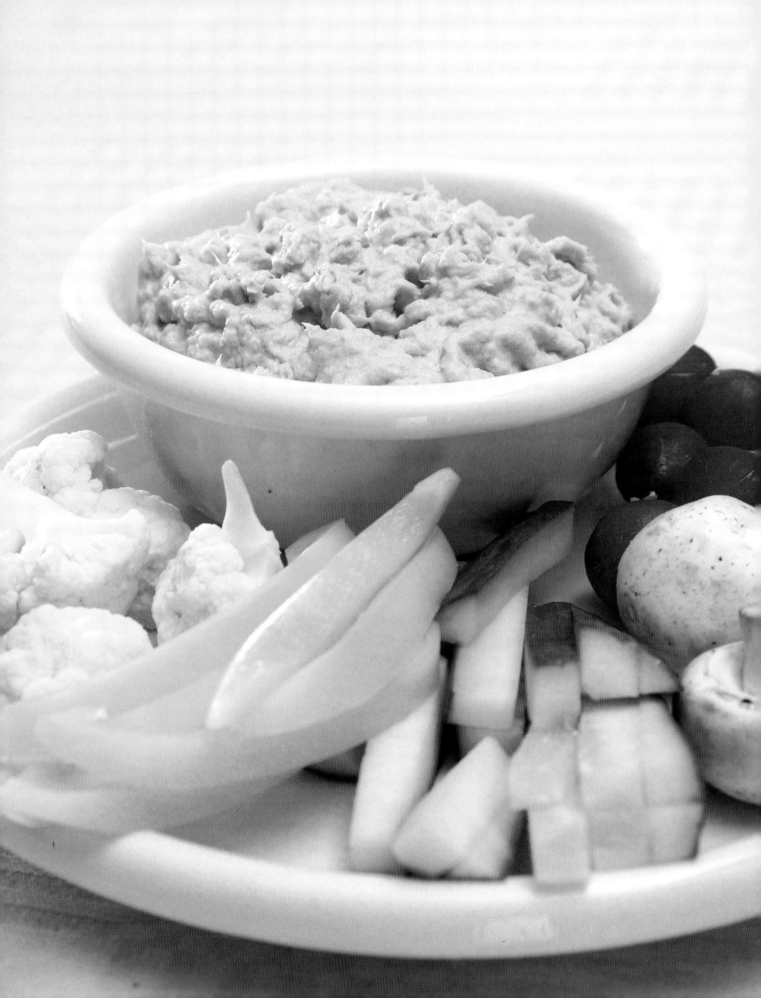

Tuna Dip with Vegetable Crudités

Quick and Easy

This dip will keep in the refrigerator for up to 3 days. It is a good idea to have vegetable crudités in the fridge to nibble on, with or without a dip. Keep them in plastic bags or in an airtight container to prevent them drying out.

Ingredients for 2

½ x 200g/7oz can tuna in
   spring water, drained
2 tsp lemon juice
50g/2oz Greek-style natural
   yoghurt
salt and freshly ground
   black pepper

Vegetables to dip, e.g.
   carrots, celery, peppers,
   mushrooms, radishes

Ingredients for 4

200g/7oz can tuna in spring
   water, drained
4 tsp lemon juice
100g/4oz Greek-style natural
   yoghurt
salt and freshly ground
   black pepper

Vegetables to dip, e.g.
   carrots, celery, peppers,
   mushrooms, radishes

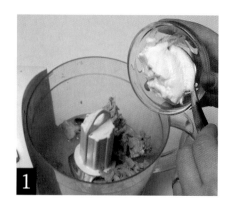

1 Place the tuna, lemon juice, yoghurt and seasoning in a food processor and blend until smooth.

2 Transfer to a serving dish.

3 Prepare the vegetables by cutting into bite-size pieces or sticks, as necessary. Serve with the dip.

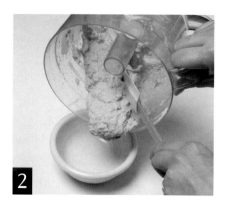

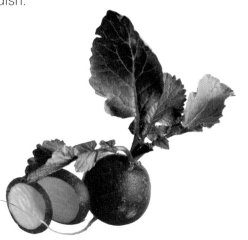

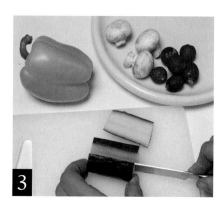

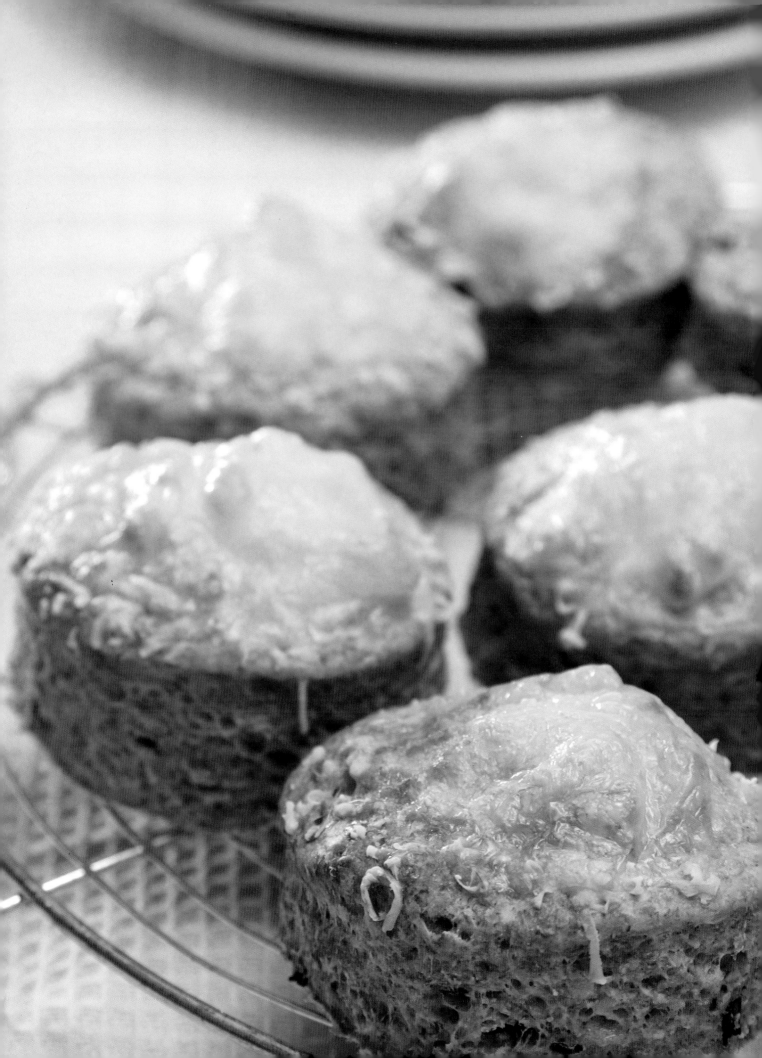

Wholemeal Scones

Serve warm, plain or spread with a little low-fat cream cheese.

Ingredients for 3-4

75g/3oz plain wholemeal
   flour
½ tsp baking powder
25g/1oz butter or sunflower
   margarine
50g/2oz reduced-fat Cheddar
   cheese, grated
1 tbsp fresh chives, snipped
1-2 tbsp skimmed or semi-
   skimmed milk, plus extra
   for brushing

Ingredients for 6-8

175g/6oz plain wholemeal
   flour
1 tsp baking powder
50g/2oz butter or sunflower
   margarine
100g/4 oz reduced-fat
   Cheddar cheese, grated
2 tbsp fresh chives, snipped
2-3 tbsp skimmed or semi-
   skimmed milk, plus extra
   for brushing

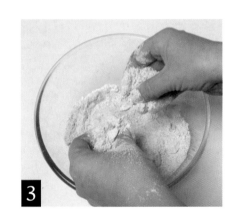

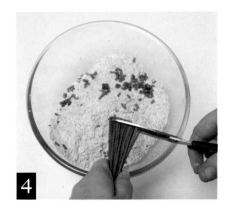

1 Preheat oven to 200°C/400°F/gas mark 6.

2 Place the flour and baking powder in a mixing bowl and stir to mix.

3 Rub in the fat until the mixture resembles fine breadcrumbs.

4 Stir in most of the cheese and chives. Add enough milk to bring the mixture together to form a soft dough.

5 Roll out the dough to about 2cm/¾in thick and cut out 7.5cm/3in scones using a round cookie cutter. Place on a lightly greased baking sheet. Re-roll the dough as required.

6 Brush the tops with a little extra milk and sprinkle the remaining cheese on top. Bake for 20 minutes or until risen and golden. Serve warm.

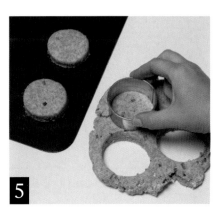

Carrot & Cheese Filo Parcels

Freezer Friendly

These tasty little filo nibbles will keep in a cool place for a day or two and freeze well. If using from frozen, thaw at room temperature. Serve hot or cold.

Ingredients for 8

15g/½oz rice noodles
50g/2oz carrots, grated
50g/2oz low-fat cream cheese
25g/1oz salted peanuts, chopped
2 sheets filo pastry
about 2 tsp olive oil
½ tsp sesame seeds

Ingredients for 18

25g/1oz rice noodles
100g/4oz carrots, grated
100g/4oz low-fat cream cheese
50g/2oz salted peanuts, chopped
4 sheets filo pastry
about 4 tsp olive oil
1 tsp sesame seeds

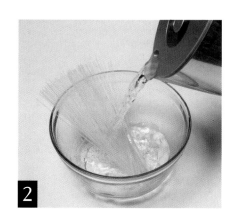

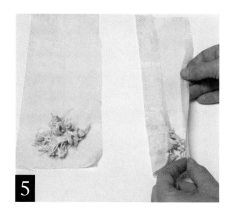

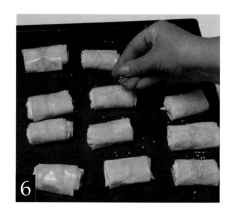

1 Preheat the oven to 200°C/400°F/gas mark 6.

2 Put the noodles in a heat-proof bowl and pour boiling water over them to cover. Allow to stand for 5 minutes, drain and snip into short lengths.

3 Put the noodles, carrots, cheese and peanuts in a bowl and mix well.

4 Place a sheet of filo on the work surface and brush with oil, then cut into 3 long rectangles.

5 Put a small amount of the carrot filling at one end of a piece of filo. Fold in the edges, then roll up.

6 Place on a baking sheet and repeat until all the pastry and filling has been used.

7 Brush the tops with a little oil and sprinkle with sesame seeds. Bake for 15 minutes until crisp and golden.

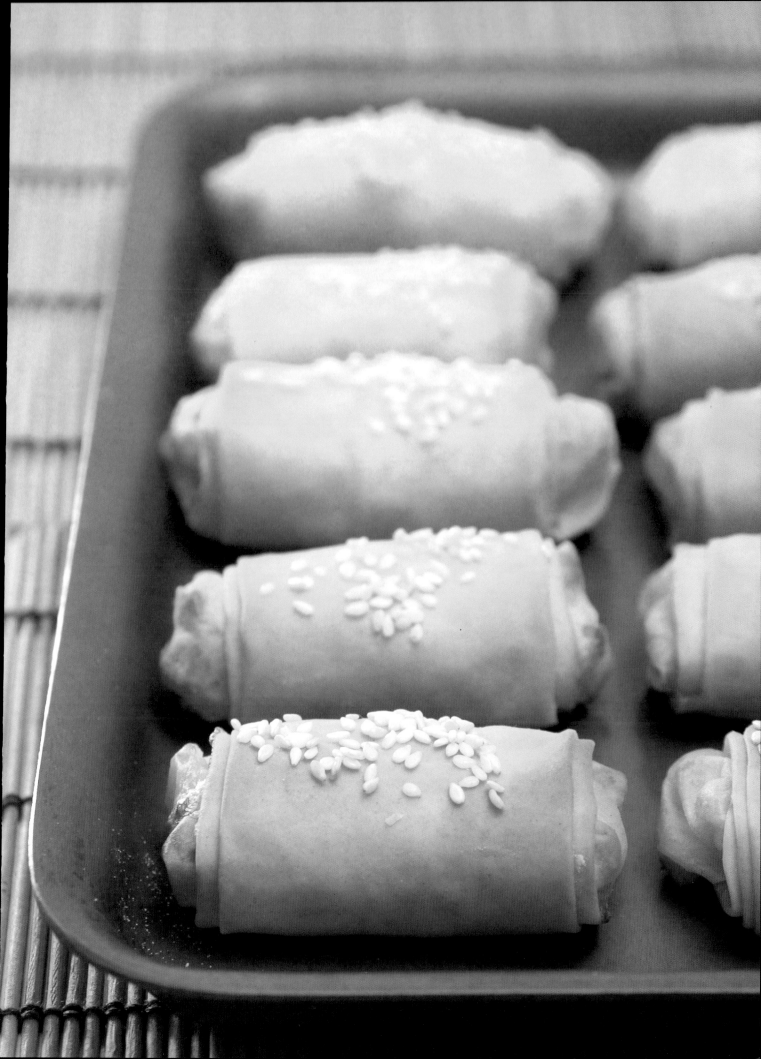

Honey Roasted Nuts

While nuts do have a relatively high fat content, they also contain fat soluble vitamins vital for good health. They are, therefore, much better to nibble on than other high-fat snacks such as chocolate or crisps, but do not be tempted to eat too many. The honey will also satisfy those with a sweet tooth.

Ingredients for 4

1 tbsp clear honey
1 tsp tamari or soy sauce
¼ tsp ground ginger
pinch of ground chilli powder
100g/4oz cashews or
    blanched almonds
25g/1oz raisins
25g/1oz no-soak dried
    apricots, chopped

Ingredients for 8

2 tbsp clear honey
2 tsp tamari or soy sauce
½ tsp ground ginger
pinch of ground chilli powder
225g/8oz cashews or
    blanched almonds
50g/2oz raisins
50g/2oz no-soak dried
    apricots, chopped

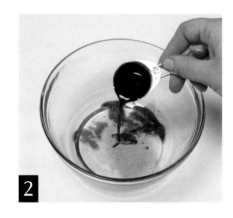

1 Preheat the oven to 170°C/325°F/gas mark 3. Lightly oil a baking sheet.

2 Mix together the honey, tamari or soy sauce and spices.

3 Stir in the nuts and toss until well coated.

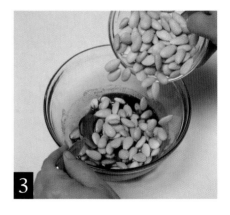

4 Tip on to the prepared baking sheet and spread into a single layer.

5 Roast for about 25 minutes, stirring occasionally. Allow to cool. Break up and mix with the dried fruit before serving.

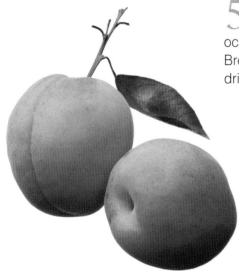

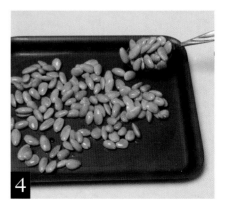

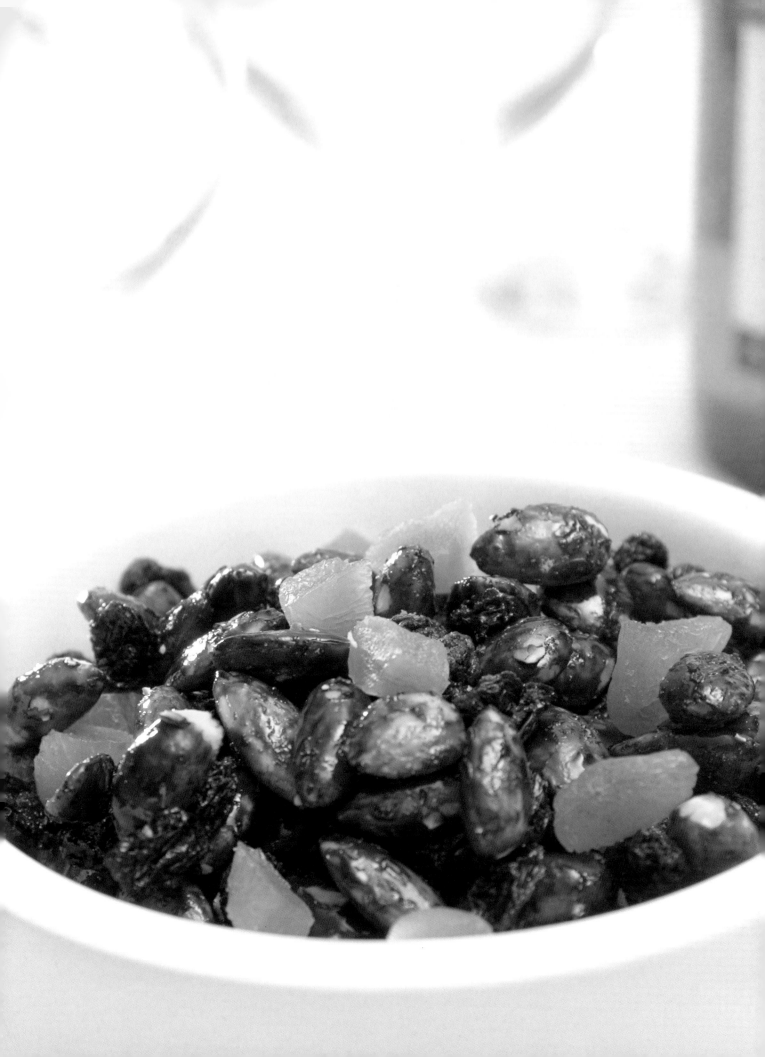

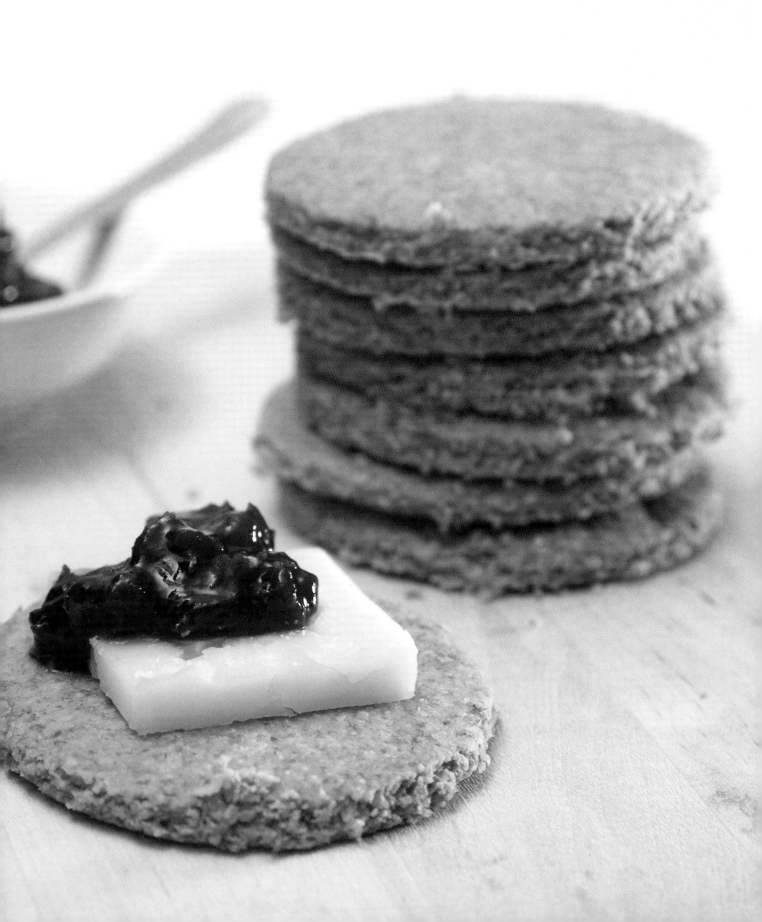

Oat Cakes

Serve these low-fat, savoury biscuits with a little low-fat cheese and pickle. They will keep in an airtight container for up to 2 weeks.

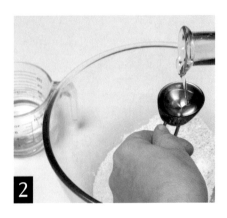

Ingredients for 6

50g/2oz fine oatmeal
25g/1oz plain wholemeal flour
½ tsp bicarbonate of soda
½ tsp caster sugar
pinch of salt
2 tbsp sunflower oil
about 2 tbsp boiling water

Ingredients for 12

100g/4oz fine oatmeal
50g/2oz plain wholemeal flour
1 tsp bicarbonate of soda
1 tsp caster sugar
pinch of salt
4 tbsp sunflower oil
2-3 tbsp boiling water

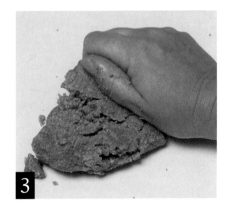

1 Preheat the oven to 180°C/350°F/gas mark 4.

2 Place the oatmeal, flour, bicarbonate of soda, sugar and salt in a mixing bowl. Stir in the oil and enough water to mix to a slightly sticky, soft dough.

3 Turn out on to a lightly floured surface and knead until the dough is no longer sticky.

4 Roll out the dough between two sheets of cling wrap until 3mm/⅛in thick and cut out 7.5cm/3in rounds with a cookie cutter. Place on lightly greased baking trays and bake for 15–20 minutes.

5 Transfer to a wire rack to cool.

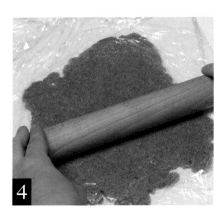

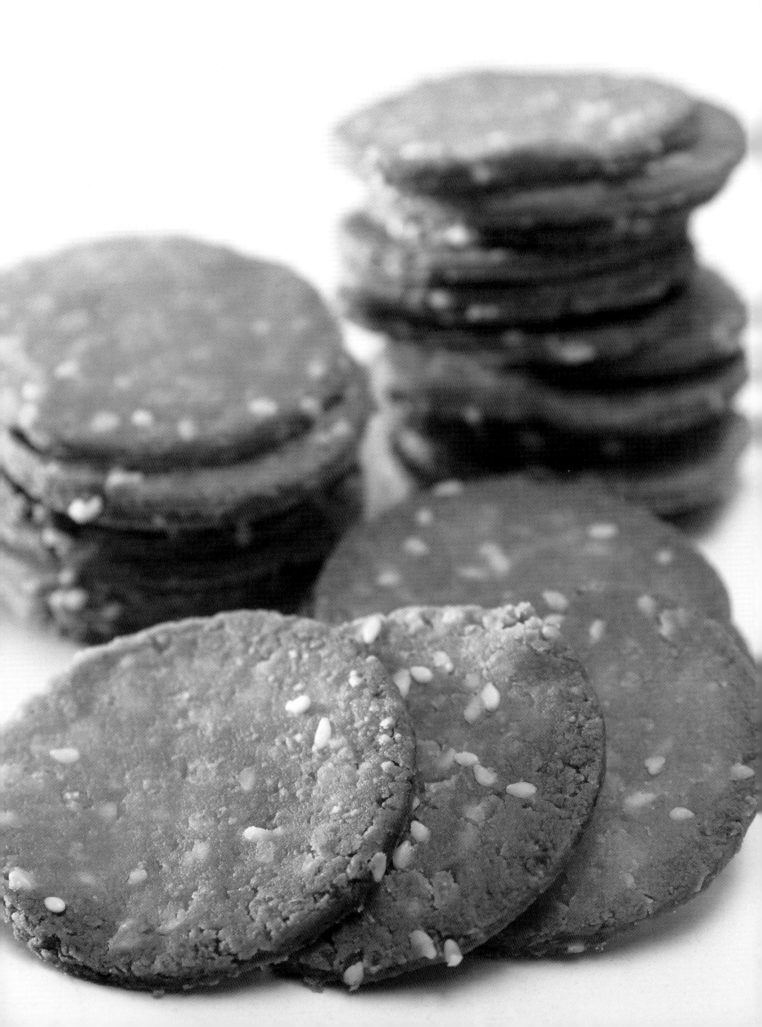

Rice Bites

These low-fat savoury biscuits are chewy, yet very morish.

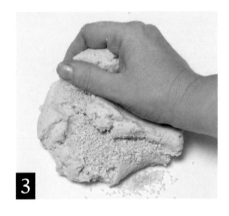

Makes 12

50g/2oz rice flour
50g/2oz cooked brown
    basmati rice
1 tbsp sunflower oil
2 tbsp water
1 tsp tamari or soy sauce
1-2 tsp sesame seeds

Makes 24

100g/4oz rice flour
100g/4oz cooked brown
    basmati rice
2 tbsp sunflower oil
4 tbsp water
2 tsp tamari or soy sauce
1 tbsp sesame seeds

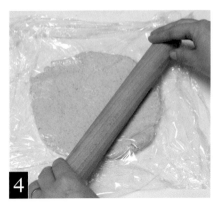

1 Preheat the oven to 190°C/375°F/gas mark 5.

2 Place all the ingredients except the sesame seeds in a food processor and blend.

3 Transfer to a bowl and mix in the sesame seeds.

4 Roll out to about 3mm/⅛in thick. If it is difficult to roll, place it between two sheets of cling wrap.

5 Using a cookie cutter, cut out 5cm/2in circles.

6 Place on a lightly oiled baking sheet and bake for 15 minutes until crisp and golden.

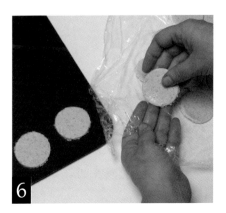

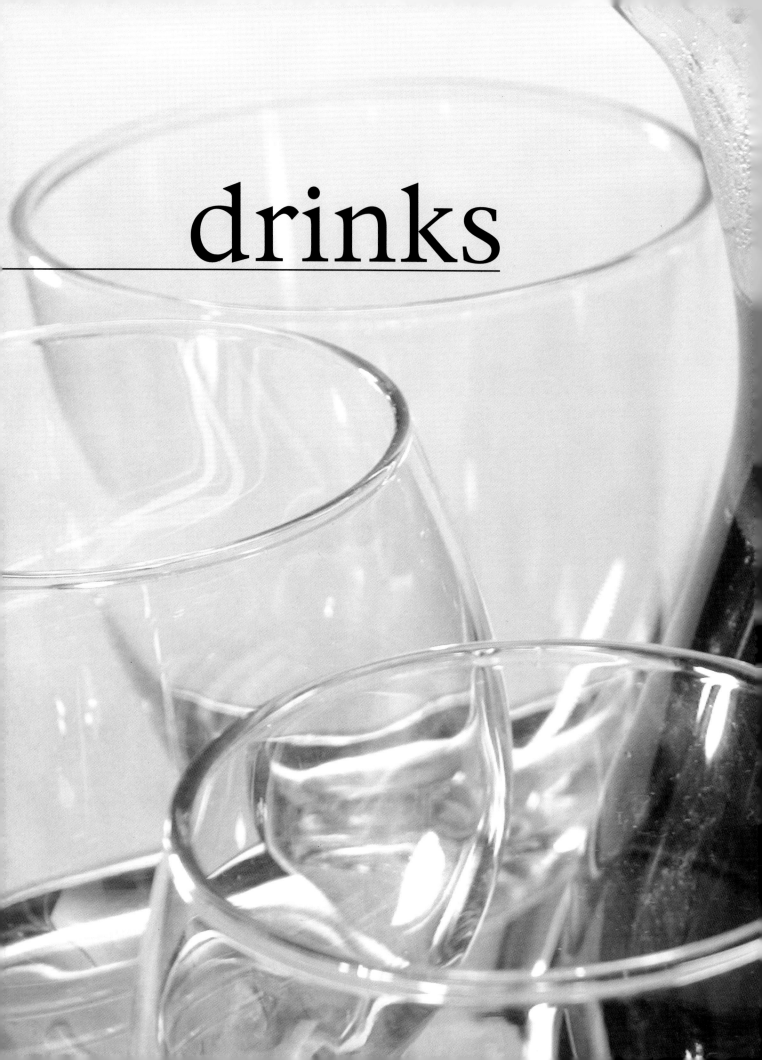

drinks

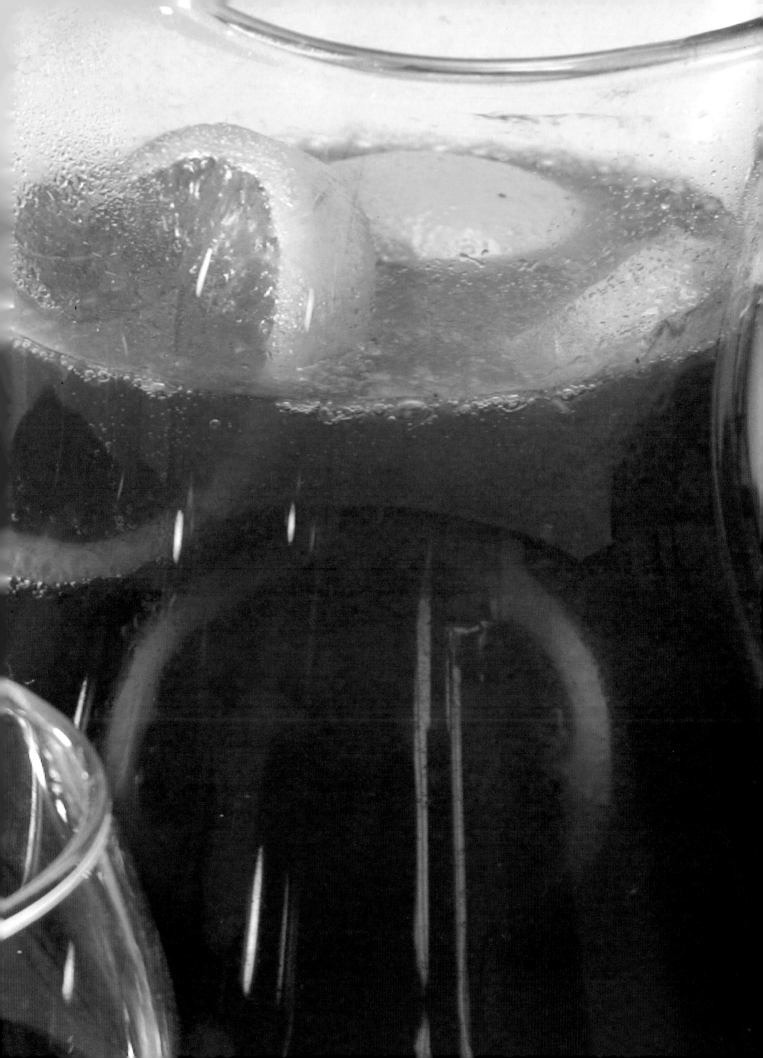

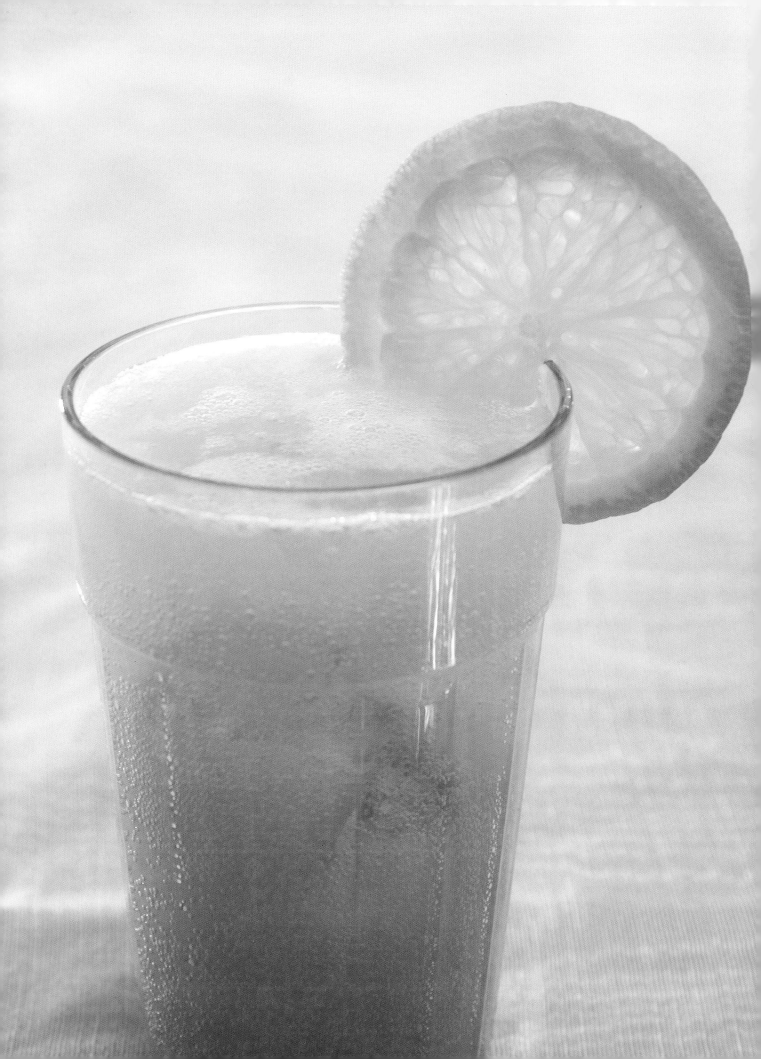

Peach, Cranberry & Orange Fizz

Easy Entertaining

This is a versatile drink that I serve at barbeques in the summer and also as a non-alcoholic festive drink at Christmas.

Serves 4-6

200g/7oz can peaches in natural juice
150ml/¼pt unsweetened orange juice
150ml/¼pt cranberry juice drink
ice
300ml/½pt sparkling mineral water
orange slices to decorate

Serves 6-8

400g/14oz can peaches in natural juice
300ml/½pt unsweetened orange juice
300ml/½pt cranberry juice drink
ice
600ml/1pt sparkling mineral water
orange slices to decorate

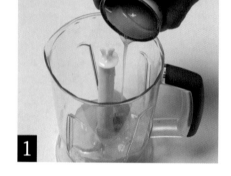

1 Place the peaches in a liquidiser and blend until smooth.

2 Mix with the orange juice and cranberry drink.

3 Divide the ice between glasses and pour juice over it.

4 Top up with mineral water.

5 Decorate with the orange slices.

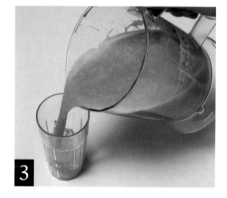

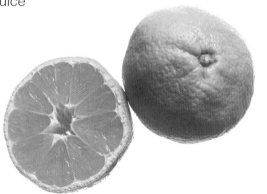

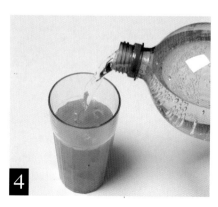

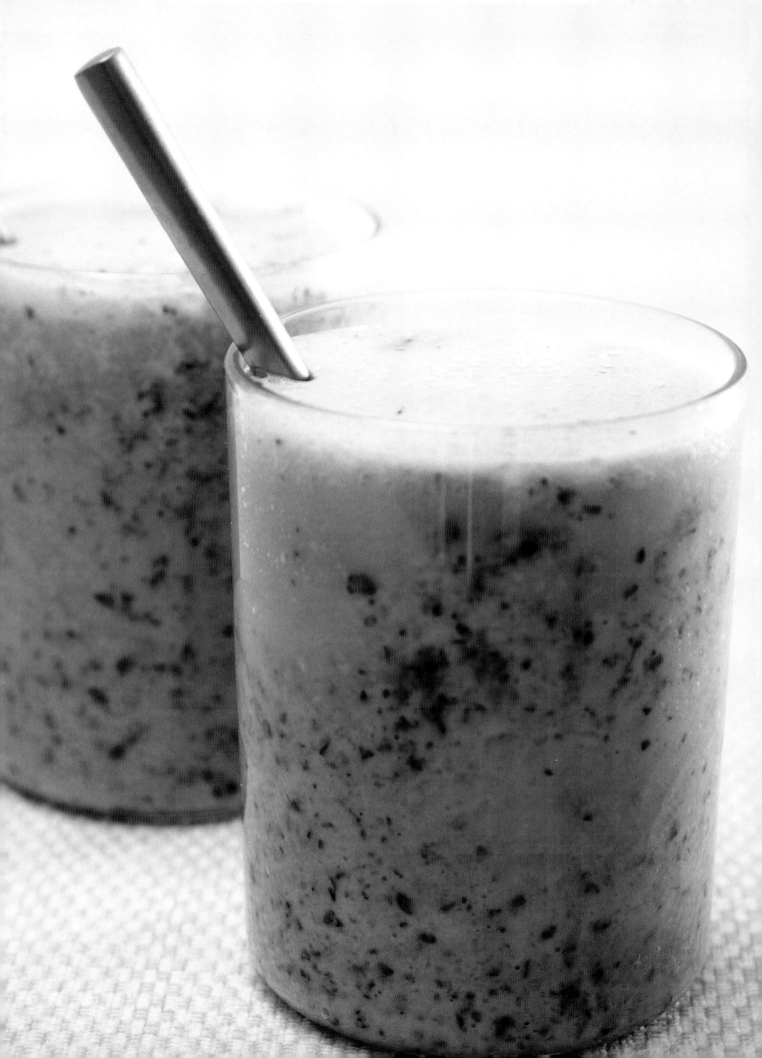

Blueberry Yoghurt Smoothie

A great way to get one of the five portions of fresh fruit and vegetables you should be consuming each day.

Ingredients for 2

100g/4oz blueberries
150g/5oz low-fat natural
    yoghurt
1 tbsp honey
ice
150ml/¼pt sparkling mineral
    water

Ingredients for 4

225g/8oz blueberries
300g/10½oz low-fat natural
    yoghurt
2 tbsp honey
ice
300ml/½pt sparkling mineral
    water

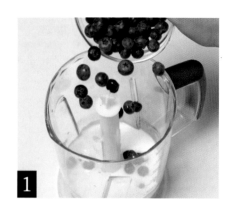

1 Place the blueberries, yoghurt and honey in a liquidiser and blend until frothy.

2 Put ice into 2 (4) glasses.

3 Divide the yoghurt drink between the 2 (4) glasses.

4 Top up with mineral water and stir before serving.

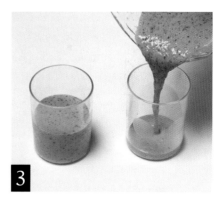

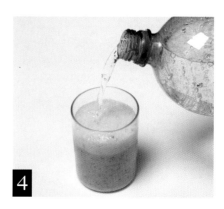

Ginger Apple Punch

Quick and Easy

A refreshing summer drink.

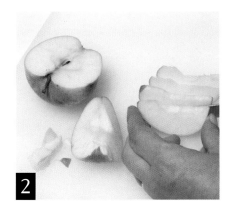

2

Ingredients for 2

**150ml/¼pt clear
   unsweetened apple juice**
1 tsp grated root ginger
1 small eating apple
ice
**300ml/½pt low cal dry
   ginger ale**

Ingredients for 4

**300ml/½pt clear
   unsweetened apple juice**
1 tbsp grated root ginger
1 eating apple
ice
**600ml/1pt low cal dry
   ginger ale**

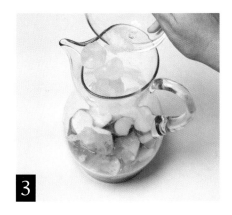

3

1 Place the apple juice in a large jug with the ginger.

2 Core and slice the apple and add to the jug.

3 Add ice.

4 Top up with ginger ale.

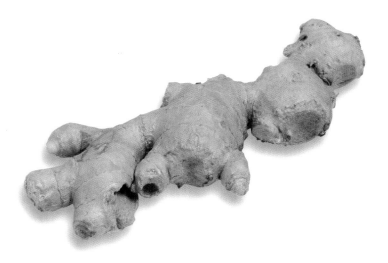

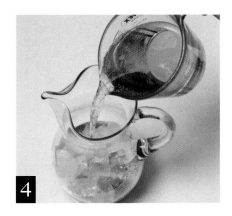

4

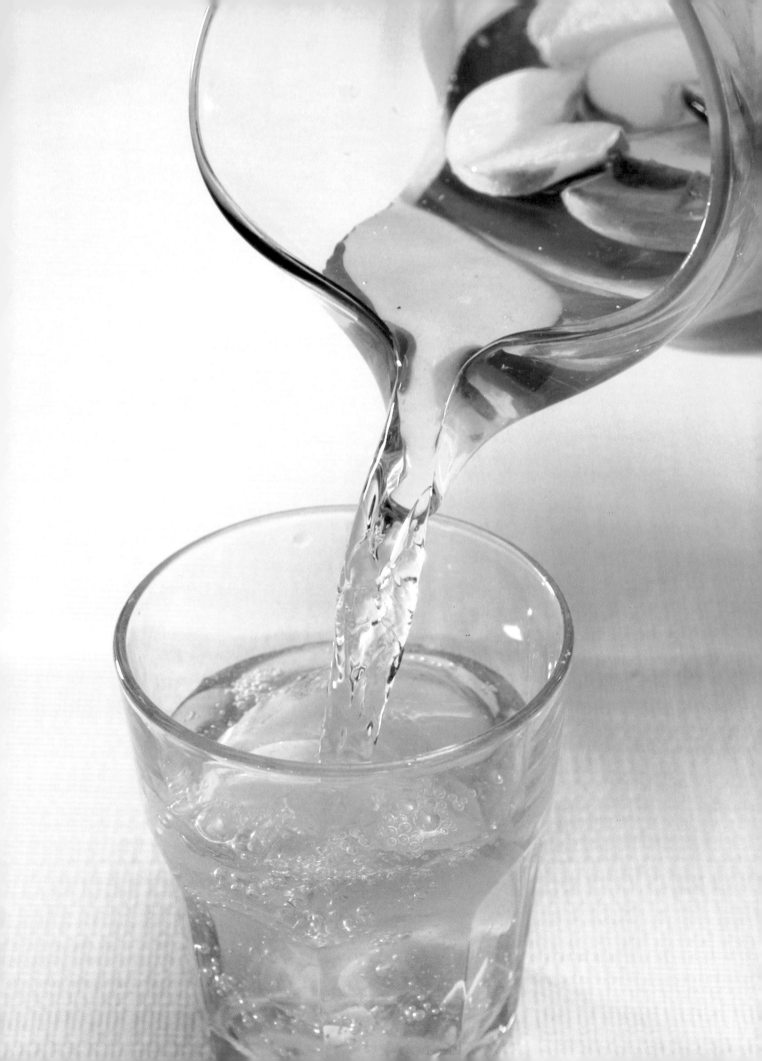

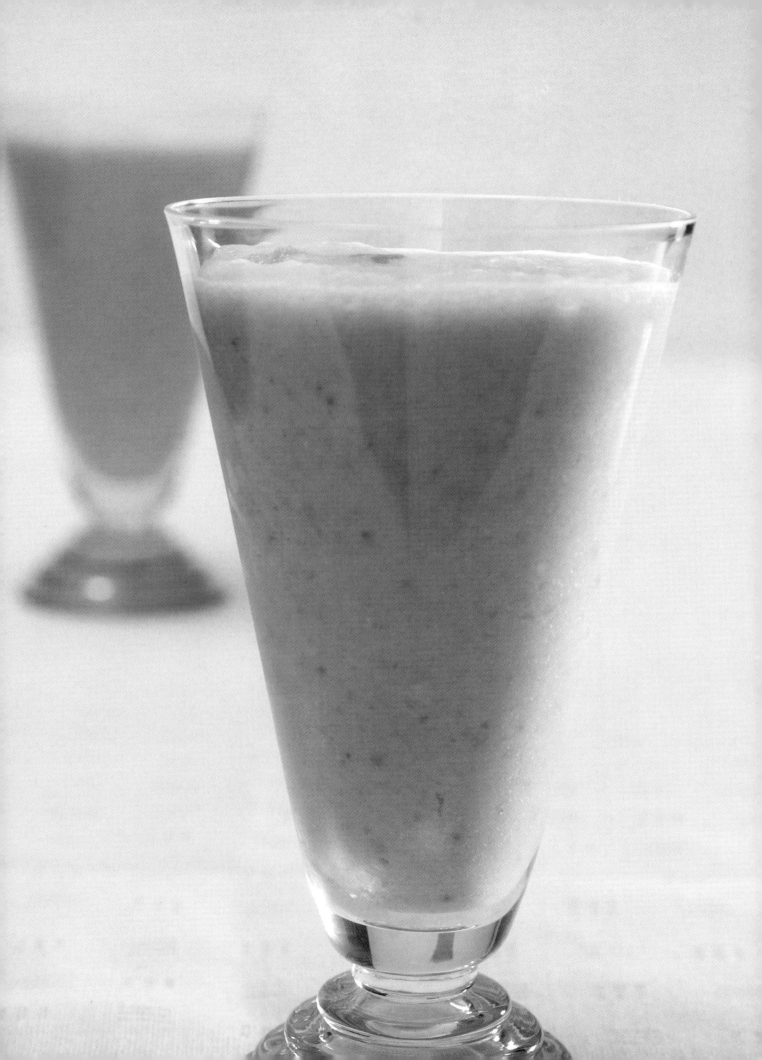

Strawberry & Banana Tofu Shake

Family Favourite

Tofu is low in fat and high in protein. Adding tofu to a milk shake is an easy way to incorporate it into the diet.

Ingredients for 2

100g/4oz strawberries, washed and hulled
1 small ripe banana
175g/6oz soft tofu
350ml/12fl oz fresh orange juice
ice to serve

Ingredients for 4

225g/8oz strawberries, washed and hulled
1 large ripe banana
350g/12oz soft tofu
750ml/1¼pt fresh orange juice
ice to serve

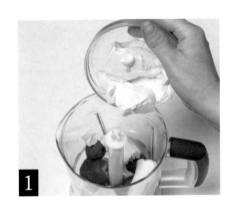

1 Place the strawberries, banana and tofu in a liquidiser and blend into a purée.

2 Add the orange juice and blend again.

3 Pour over the ice to serve.

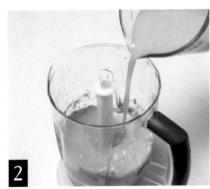

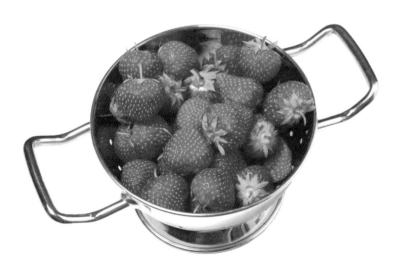

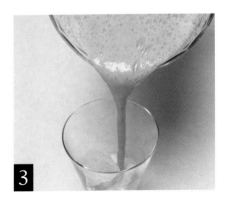

Iced Tea

Fizzy drinks are full of sugar and I do not like low-cal fizzy drinks very much, so I find iced tea a perfect refreshing drink when it's hot. You can sweeten the tea with intense sweetener instead of honey if you prefer.

Ingredients for 2

2 tsp Ceylon tea
450ml/¾pt boiling water
2 tsp clear honey
1-2 tsp lemon or lime juice
ice
lemon or lime slices to serve

Ingredients for 4

4 tsp Ceylon tea
900ml/1½pt boiling water
4 tsp clear honey
1 tbsp lemon or lime juice
ice
lemon or lime slices to serve

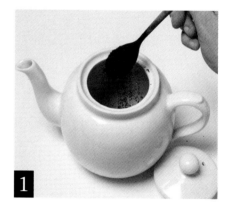

1 Place the tea in a pot and add the boiling water. Leave to infuse for 5 minutes.

2 Strain into a heatproof jug.

3 Stir in the honey and lemon or lime juice.

4 Allow to cool then cover and chill for at least 1 hour. Serve with ice and a slice of fruit if liked.

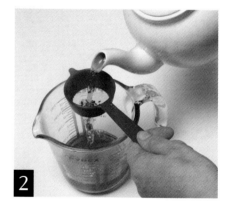

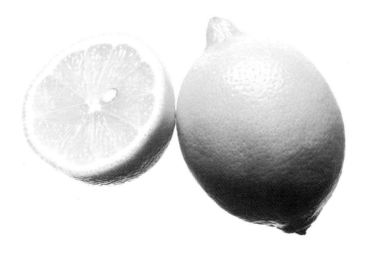

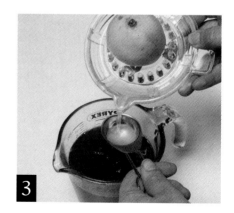

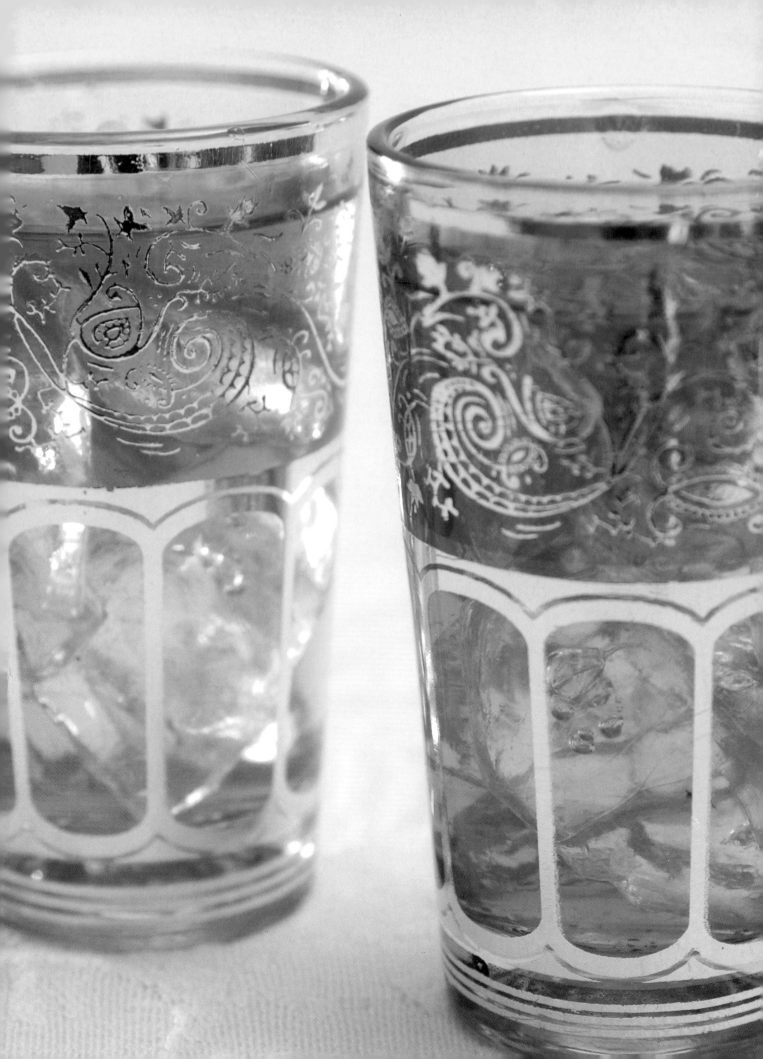

Sangria

Easy Entertaining

There is no reason why people with diabetes cannot still enjoy the occasional alcoholic drink, and this summery fruit punch is perfect for al fresco eating. Do remember that it is important to have a snack when drinking. Never drink on an empty stomach as this can lower blood glucose levels.

Ingredients for 2

350ml/12fl oz red wine
3 tbsp brandy
75ml/2½fl oz orange juice
1 small orange, sliced
1 lemon, sliced
ice
300ml/½pt diet lemonade

Ingredients for 4

75cl bottle of red wine
100ml/3½fl oz brandy
150ml/¼pt orange juice
1 orange, sliced
1 lemon, sliced
ice
600ml/1pt diet lemonade

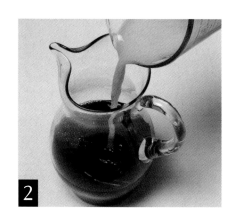

1 Pour the wine into a large jug.

2 Add the brandy and orange juice.

3 Add the fruit slices and a handful of ice.

4 Top up with lemonade

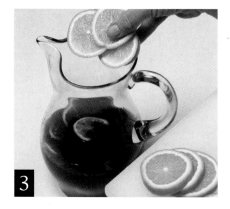

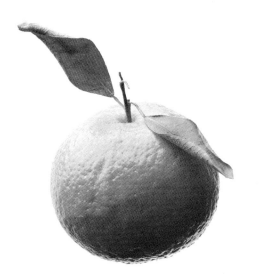

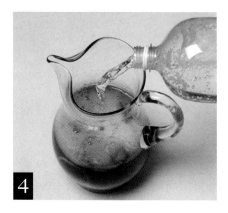

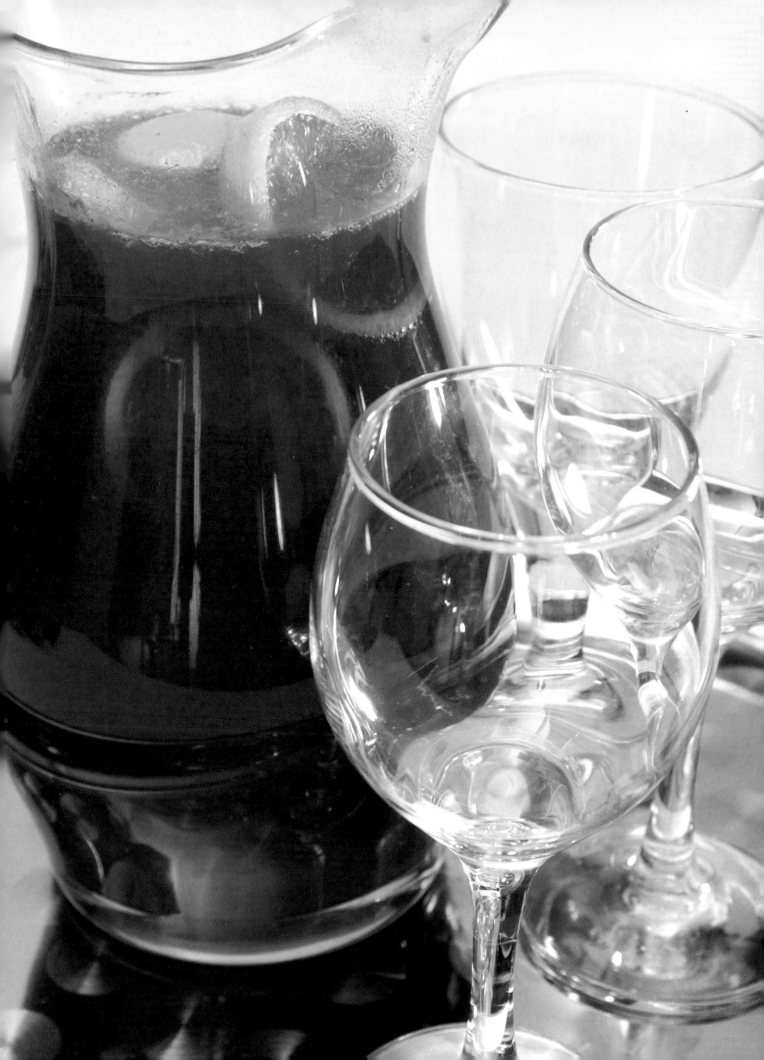

glossary

Blood glucose

The level of glucose in the bloodstream.

Carbohydrate

Carbohydrates supply most of our energy. They come in three main forms: starch, sugar and cellulose (fibre). Most of our energy intake should come from the starchy carbohydrates, such as potatoes, rice, pasta and bread.

Glucose

Glucose is a type of sugar found in carbohydrates, and is our body's main source of energy.

Glycogen

The form in which glucose is stored in the liver.

Hyperglycaemic

Occurs when blood sugars are too high.

Hypoglycaemic

Occurs when blood sugars are too low.

Insulin

The hormone that controls glucose in the bloodstream.

Pancreas

The gland that produces insulin.

Type I Diabetes

People with Type I diabetes have a severe shortage of insulin. Generally, Type I diabetes needs to be treated with regular injections of insulin and a healthy eating routine. It usually occurs in people under 40.

Type II Diabetes

This is the most common form of diabetes and accounts for 75% of people with the disease. The body makes some insulin but not enough. This form of diabetes is generally treated by a controlled diet and sometimes additional medication. Most people with Type II diabetes are overweight and over 40 years of age. However, with the increase of obesity more and more people are being diagnosed with Type II diabetes at an earlier age.

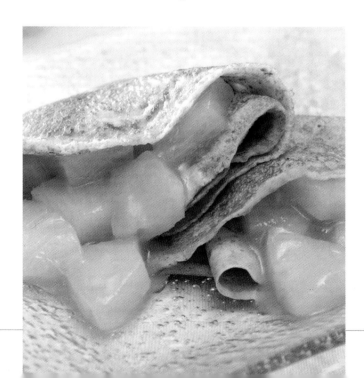

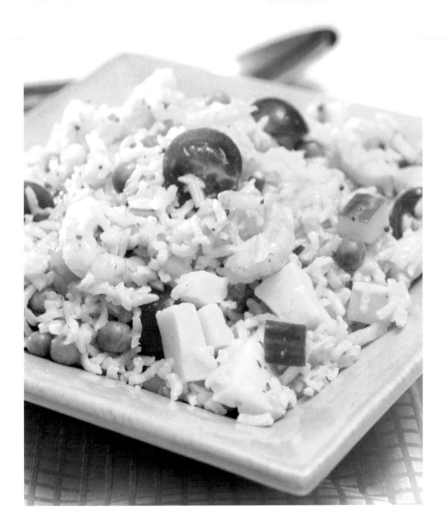

information

Further information can be obtained from:

Diabetes UK
10 Parkway
London
NW1 7AA

Tel: 020 7424 1000
Fax 020 7424 1001

Website: www.diabetes.org.uk

Diabetes UK Careline: 0845 1202960

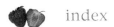

index

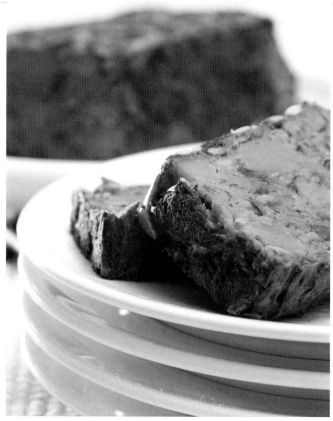

credits & acknowledgements

Thank you to Louise Blair, consultant food writer to Diabetes UK, for checking all my copy and ensuring that all the recipes follow the healthy eating guidelines recommended for people with diabetes. Also thanks for her helpful advice in producing this book.

Thanks also to Richard, James, William, Colin and Paul for being willing guinea pigs tasting the recipes, and for giving their honest opinions – which I am glad to say were mostly positive.

Thanks to Harrison Fisher and Co (www.premiercutlery.co.uk) for supplying the knives and some of the small kitchen utensils used for the step-by-step pictures. Also thanks to Magimix whose food processor has well and truly earned its place on my kitchen worktop, making light work of the soups and some of the other dishes in this book.